DATE DUE

JUL 27 2012	
APR 0 8 2013	
SEP 1 7 2015	

Mild Cognitive Impairment and
Early Alzheimer's Disease

Mild Cognitive Impairment and
Early Alzheimer's Disease
Detections and Diagnosis

JEFFREY M. BURNS MD
Director of the Alzheimer and Memory Center and
the Alzheimer Disease Clinical Research Program
Department of Neurology, University of Kansas School of Medicine
Kansas City, Kansas, UNITED STATES

JOHN C. MORRIS MD
Friedman Distinguished Professor of Neurology
Professor of Pathology and Immunology
Professor of Physical Therapy
Director, Alzheimer's Disease Research Center
Director, Center for Aging, Washington University, St. Louis, Missouri, UNITED STATES

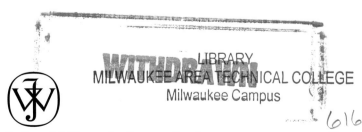

John Wiley & Sons, Ltd

Copyright © 2008   John Wiley & Sons Ltd, The Atrium, Southern Gate, Chichester,
                          West Sussex PO19 8SQ, England

                          Telephone   (+44) 1243 779777

Email (for orders and customer service enquiries): cs-books@wiley.co.uk
Visit our Home Page on www.wileyeurope.com or www.wiley.com

Other Wiley Editorial Offices

John Wiley & Sons Inc., 111 River Street, Hoboken, NJ 07030, USA

Jossey-Bass, 989 Market Street, San Francisco, CA 94103-1741, USA

Wiley-VCH Verlag GmbH, Boschstr. 12, D-69469 Weinheim, Germany

John Wiley & Sons Australia Ltd, 33 Park Road, Milton, Queensland 4064, Australia

John Wiley & Sons (Asia) Pte Ltd, 2 Clementi Loop #02-01, Jin Xing Distripark, Singapore 129809

John Wily & Sons Canada Ltd, 6045 Freemont Blvd, Mississauga, Ontario, L5R 4J3, Canada

Wiley also publishes its books in a variety of electronic formats. Some content that appears in print may not be
available in electronic books.

Library of Congress Cataloging-in-Publication Data

Burns, Jeffrey M. (Jeffrey Murray)
   Early diagnosis and treatment of mild cognitive impairment / Jeffrey M.
Burns, John C. Morris.
      p. ; cm.
   Includes bibliographical references and index.
   ISBN 978-0-470-31936-9 (cloth : alk. paper)   1. Cognition disorders
in old age—Diagnosis.   2. Cognition disorders in old age—Treatment.
3. Presenile dementia—Diagnosis.   4. Presenile dementia—Treatment.
I. Morris, John C., 1948- II. Title.
   [DNLM: 1. Cognition Disorders.   2. Aged.   3. Alzheimer Disease.   4.
Dementia. WT 150 B9675e 2008]
   RC553.C64B87 2008
   616.8075—dc22

                                                                              2008007182

British Library Cataloguing in Publication Data

A catalogue record for this book is available from the British Library

ISBN   9780470319369

Produced from Quark files supplied by Nova professional Media Ltd.
This book is printed on acid-free paper
Printed and bound in Spain by Grafos SA., Barcelona

Contents

1   **Introduction 1**
What is mild cognitive impairment? **3**
   Epidemiological studies of MCI **5**

The border zone between aging and dementia: cognitive and
neuropathological changes **10**
   Aging and cognitive performance **11**

2   **Neuropathology of Alzheimer's disease, non-demented
aging and MCI 17**
Histopathological features **17**
   Plaques **18**
   Neurofibrillary pathology **18**
   Neuronal loss **19**
   Topography of neuropathological changes **22**
   Neuropathological AD diagnosis **24**

Neuropathology of aging **27**

Neuropathology of MCI **31**

Does a subset of MCI patients actually have early Alzheimer's
disease? **32**
   Clinical studies **32**
   Neuroimaging **32**

3   **Detecting and diagnosing MCI and early AD 35**
Early detection **35**

Recognition of MCI and early AD **36**
   Informant-based history **39**
   Neurological examination **41**
   Laboratory and radiological evaluation **42**
   Psychometric/mental status testing **44**

Dementia-screening instruments **45**
   Mini-mental state examination **45**
   Clock-drawing test **46**
   Seven-minute screen **48**

Dementia staging instruments **49**
   CDR **49**
   Global deterioration scale **50**

4   **Etiology of MCI: differential diagnosis 53**
"Worried-well" **53**

Depression **54**

Other etiologies **55**

Neurodegenerative dementias **55**
   Overlap disorders **58**
   Dementia with Lewy bodies **58**
   Vascular dementia **59**
   Frontotemporal lobar dementias **60**

Identifying the subset of MCI that is AD **65**

5   **Treatment of MCI and dementia 69**
MCI **69**
   The case for early treatment **69**
   Non-pharmacological treatment **71**

Dementia therapy **73**
   Approved therapies **73**
      Cholinergic hypothesis **73**
      Cholinesterase inhibitors **75**
      Donepezil **77**
      Rivastigmine **78**
      Galantamine **79**
      Memantine **79**

   Agents under investigation for AD treatment and
   prevention **81**
      Vitamin E and selegiline **81**
      Estrogen **82**
      Anti-inflammatory agents **83**
      Cholesterol-reducing agents **84**
      Chelation therapy **84**

6 **Future therapeutic and diagnostic strategies 85**
Amyloid hypothesis **85**
   Secretase inhibitors **87**
   Amyloid vaccine **88**
Potential biomarkers **89**
   CSF biomarkers **90**
      CSF amyloid beta (Aβ) **91**
      CSF tau **91**
      CSF sulfatide **92**
      CSF markers of inflammation **93**
      CSF markers of oxidative stress **93**
   Serum biomarkers **94**
Structural imaging **95**
Functional neuroimaging **96**
   PET and SPECT **97**
   Functional MRI (fMRI) **98**
   Imaging amyloid **100**
Genetic testing **101**
   Early-onset familial AD **102**
      Amyloid precursor protein **102**
      Presenilin genes **103**
   Late-onset AD **103**
      Apolipoprotein E **104**

7 **Case studies 105**
Case report 1: MCI as early-stage Alzheimer's disease **105**
   Comment **108**
Case report 2: Diagnosis of dementia prior to impairment sufficient for MCI **110**
   Comment **113**
Case report 3: Memory complaints associated with non-demented aging **118**
   Comment **121**

References 123
Index 143

Introduction

The past two decades have been marked by the introduction of
effective symptomatic therapies for Alzheimer's disease (AD),
discovery of causative mutations that result in early-onset forms
of the disorder, development of animal models of AD, and the
increased ability to detect the disease clinically in its earliest
symptomatic stages. Discriminating the initial manifestations of AD
from the cognitive changes that accompany usual aging, however,
remains in many instances a difficult task. This diagnostic dilemma
is complicated by the increasing prevalence of AD with age, such
that perhaps as many as 50% of individuals aged 85 years or older
are affected. Distinguishing cognitive complaints of the "old old"
that reflect true aging versus those that herald a dementing disorder
such as AD becomes increasingly problematic (Figures 1.1 and 1.2).

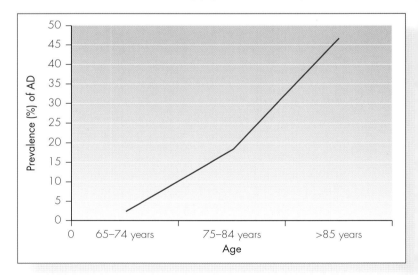

FIGURE 1.1 Prevalence of Alzheimer's disease in the aging population. The prevalence
of Alzheimer's disease increases dramatically with age and approaches 50% of those
over 85 years old.[38]

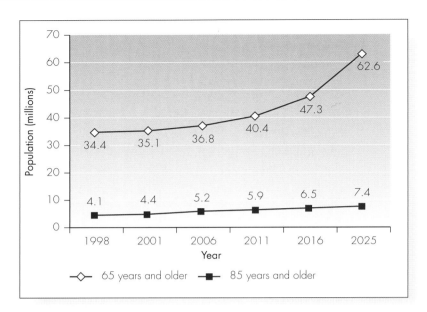

FIGURE 1.2 Population estimate for older adults in the U.S.A.: 2000 Census Bureau estimate. The US Census Bureau projects the population of 65 years and older will increase dramatically by the year 2025 (middle-series estimates). The 85 years and older group is the fastest growing segment of the population.

The term "mild cognitive impairment" (MCI)[12] has been proposed to represent the border zone between aging and dementia. It characterizes individuals with cognitive changes beyond those typical for truly healthy aging but that fall short of what currently is recognized as dementia. Its importance comes from the assumption that embedded within the MCI condition are many individuals with prodromal or incipient dementia. Identifying these individuals, as opposed to those with MCI who do not have an underlying dementing illness, will allow the earliest symptomatic stages of dementia to be better recognized and treated. MCI has been estimated to affect 10–17% of the elderly population.[13,14] Although not all MCI individuals will progress to further stages of cognitive impairment, many individuals considered to have MCI already may have very mild dementia. Thus, the true prevalence of AD may be much greater than is currently appreciated.

Identifying that subset of individuals who will go on to develop frank dementia or AD is the focus of intense interest for management and treatment purposes. The importance of diagnosing dementia early has increased with the advent of approved symptomatic therapy for mild to moderate AD. Accurate and early recognition of dementia also enables patient autonomy in advance directives and other life decisions, and aids families in planning for care giving and other adaptations before a crisis is reached. Finally, potential disease-modifying agents under development, which may halt progression or even prevent AD and other dementing illnesses, likely will be most effective when initiated as early in the disease course as possible.

The purpose of this monograph is to describe cognitive changes with age, the earliest detectable stages of AD, and the relation of these conditions to MCI. This monograph will address current concepts in MCI, including its definition, prevalence, evaluation, management, and outcomes. In particular, it will examine the relationship of MCI to AD, by far the most common dementing disorder in late life, and assist practicing physicians in the identification of that subset of MCI patients who will progress to recognized AD.

What is mild cognitive impairment?

The term "mild cognitive impairment" is one of many that have been introduced to characterize the boundary of aging and dementia.[12,13,15–17] MCI was specifically intended to capture those patients destined to develop dementia.[12] The cognitive changes associated with MCI are assumed to be pathological and not a normal occurrence with aging,[19] rather than an inevitable part of the aging process (as intended for the diagnostic entities, "benign senescent forgetfulness"[15] and "age-associated memory impairment"[16]).

The symptomatic onset of AD is insidious. AD almost always begins with a period of subtle cognitive impairments that do not interfere considerably with daily functioning. Thus, the border-zone between aging and dementia that is characterized by MCI includes individuals in a prodromal stage of AD that occurs prior to the diagnosis of overt dementia. MCI, however, is a heterogeneous condition. While MCI captures some individuals with the earliest symptoms of AD or other forms of dementia (i.e. vascular dementia, frontotemporal dementia, dementia with Lewy bodies), it may also encompass many different non-progressive conditions. These include static cognitive impairment, the "worried-well" state, and reversible forms of cognitive dysfunction such as those related to depression, medications, or medical illnesses (Table 1.1).

TABLE 1.1 Proposed MCI etiologies

Dementia prodrome
- Alzheimer's disease
- Vascular dementia
- Frontotemporal dementia
- Dementia with Lewy bodies

Static cognitive impairment

"Worried-well"
- Cognitive complaints without cognitive impairment; often related to anxiety

Reversible cognitive dysfunction
- Depression
- Medical illnesses (i.e. thyroid dysfunction, vitamin B12 deficiency)

Structural brain disease
- Cerebrovascular disease

Cognitive effects of medications (e.g. anticholinergics)

No consensus yet exists on a set of rigorous, standardized criteria for MCI. Commonly used features for the diagnosis of MCI include (1) evidence of cognitive impairment, (2) preservation of general cognition and functional abilities, and (3) absence of diagnosed dementia. By far the most studied subset of MCI is amnestic MCI[20] (also termed MCI of the Alzheimer type[21]). Memory complaints, rather than deficits in other cognitive domains, are the hallmark of amnestic MCI. The most commonly used operational criteria for identifying amnestic MCI[22] require: (1) memory complaint, preferably corroborated by an informant; (2) memory performance 1.5 SD (standard deviations) below age- and education-appropriate norms (e.g. on a prose-recall measure); (3) normal general cognitive ability as indicated by a score of 24 or above on the MMSE (mini-mental state examination); (4) sufficiently preserved competence in activities of daily living so that dementia is not diagnosed; and (5) a CDR (clinical dementia rating) of 0.5, where 0 = no dementia and 1 = mild dementia. These criteria provide a starting point for studies of this condition, and variations are currently being adapted to identify individuals for multi-center trials of agents that may delay "conversion" of MCI to AD (Table 1.2).

Epidemiological studies of MCI

Prevalence estimates for MCI demonstrate considerable variability, ranging from 2.8% to as high as 23.4%.[1,23–27] This wide variability is due to differences in MCI definitions, study design (retrospective versus prospective), and the sample studied (referral-based versus population-based).[28] For instance, retrospectively applying MCI criteria (memory impairment 1 SD below the average of their cohort, but with intact activities of daily living (ADL) and normal general cognitive function) to a population-based sample of individuals 60 years of age and older led to MCI prevalence estimates of 3%; however, many subjects initially classified as having MCI were later classified as normal.[24] Another population-based study, defining MCI as impairment in visual memory with normal general cognitive function (MMSE score not < 1 SD below the mean), found the prevalence of MCI to be 2.8%. A higher estimate was found in the Canadian Study of Health and Aging, where the reported prevalence rate for cognitive impairment without dementia (defined by modified mini-mental state score < 78, while not meeting study criteria for dementia) was 16.8%.[13] Another study found that

TABLE 1.2 Definitions of mild cognitive impairment. In its broadest form (A), MCI represents a heterogeneous condition including early dementia of multiple types (i.e. vascular MCI), reversible causes of multiple types (i.e. depression), the "worried well", and long-standing cognitive problems. Amnestic MCI (B) was conceptualized as the earliest stage of Alzheimer's disease. Its operational definition (C) may identify a less heterogeneous population and has, in practice, come to represent those at risk of early Alzheimer's disease.

A) MCI
1. Evidence of cognitive impairment
2. Preserved general cognitive abilities
3. Not demented

B) Amnestic MCI[81]
1. Memory complaint
2. Objective memory impairment
3. Normal general cognition
4. Not demented

C) Operationalized amnestic MCI[20]
1. Memory complaint, verified by an informant
2. Memory impairment 1.5 standard deviations below normal (adjusted for age and education)
3. Normal general cognition (mini-mental state score of 24 or above)
4. Dementia not present as defined by preserved activities of daily living
5. Clinical dementia rating of 0.5

nearly 25% of community-dwelling individuals had some form of cognitive impairment.[25] The exact criteria used to define MCI and the sample to which it is applied (e.g., population-based versus referral-based) strongly influence how broadly MCI is characterized and, correspondingly, contribute to variability in results across studies.

Estimates of the risk of "conversion" from MCI to AD are also widely variable, ranging from 3.7% per annum[24] to 25% per annum in selected samples.[12,2,50] In general, individuals with MCI progress to overt AD at a rate far above the baseline dementia incidence rate of 0.2% for non-demented individuals aged 65–69 years and 3.9% for those aged 85–89 years. Thus, the risk of "conversion" to overt AD is significantly increased compared with a normal elderly population (Table 1.3).

Differences in MCI definitions and assessment techniques across studies have led to criticism of the MCI diagnostic criteria.[19,28] Currently, there is no standard neuropsychological test of memory for establishing objective evidence of memory impairment. Variable cut-off scores define when cognition is abnormal or when "normal general cognitive function" is present. Cognitive complaints may be self-reported as opposed to verified by a knowledgeable informant, an important distinction as self-reported memory complaints do not correlate with memory performance, and an informant's report is more reliable and more sensitive in detecting dementia than both cognitive test performance and the patient's self-report.[31,32] Additionally, establishing that there is interference with daily functioning is problematic, given a lack of current guidelines or diagnostic criteria. Functional deficits not routinely evident may be apparent when a knowledgeable informant is carefully and thoroughly probed.[32–36]

The widespread application of MCI criteria in a multicenter clinical-trial setting successfully identified a sample of subjects with cognitive and functional characteristics that fall between nondemented controls and AD.[37] It remains to be seen, however, whether these criteria can be effectively applied to the general population. At least two population-based studies have suggested great difficulty in applying these criteria to the general population. These population based studies reported low MCI prevalence estimates and an unstable diagnosis; many subjects initially diagnosed with MCI were later found to be normal.[23,24] Highly selected samples of MCI subjects (for instance, referred to specialized centers) appear to progress to AD at a higher rate than those subjects identified in population-based studies, while applying the MCI clinical criteria to a population-based sample may identify a more heterogeneous sample with a lower proportion progressing to more overt symptoms of AD. Thus, the application of MCI criteria to a population-based sample may be problematic.

TABLE 1.3 Risk of developing Alzheimer's disease in individuals with MCI.
Longitudinal estimates of risk of conversion from MCI to AD are widely variable, likely a result of discrepant MCI criteria and samples studied. Overall, however, MCI cohorts progress to AD at a rate

Study	Annual conversion rate	MCI subjects (no.)	Follow-up period	Overall conversion to AD	Other observations
Bennet et al. 2002[18]	7.6%	211	4.5 years	34%	29.9% of MCI subjects died (1.7 times more likely than controls
Petersen et al. 1999[20]	12%	76	4 years	48%	80% of this cohort converted to dementia at 6 years in subsequent assessments[81]
Devanand et al. 1997[39]	16.5%	75	2.5 years	41.3%	
Flicker et al.[16] 1997[12]	25%	32	2 years	50%	
Bowen et al. 1997[29]	12%	21	4 years	48%	The 21 subjects were selected from a cohort of 811 patients with cognitive complaints (2.6%)
Tierney et al. 1996[75]	11.8%	123	2 years	23.6%	
Ritchie et al.[19] 2001[24]	3.7%	65 MCI diagnoses at 3 annual visits	3 years	11.1%	MCI diagnosis was unstable over time, with almost all subjects changing category each year
Larrieu et al.[20] 2002[23]	8.3%	58	5 years	*	Incidence of MCI in people aged 70 years and older estimated to be 1% per year. MCI group very unstable – over 2–3 years of follow-up, 6% of subjects continued to have MCI while >40% reverted to normal status

* Data not shown

far above baseline dementia incidence. This suggests that embedded within a sample of MCI individuals is a subset with the earliest cognitive changes of AD. Accurate identification of this subset of MCI patients has been demonstrated in at least one longitudinal MCI study. (Morris 2001)[72]

Ascertainment	MCI criteria
Catholic nuns, priests, and brothers of the Religious Orders Study	1. Neuropsychologist's judgment of cognitive impairment after review of cognitive testing 2. Clinician's judgment of "not demented"
Alzheimer Disease Center	1. Memory complaint 2. Normal ADLs 3. Normal general cognitive function 4. Abnormal memory testing 5. Not demented
Memory Disorders Clinic	Questionable dementia 1. Minimal evidence of cognitive impairment on clinical or neuropsychological evaluation 2. Modified MMSE >30 (range 0–57) 3. Collateral source serves as informant
Aging and Dementia Research Center	Global deterioration scale rating of 3
Alzheimer's disease registry	Neuropsychological testing reveals memory loss without impairment in other cognitive realms (judgment, abstract thinking or other higher-cortical functions)
Physician-based referral for "3-month history of memory problems interfering with function"	1. Global deterioration scale rating of 2 or 3 2. MMSE score ≥ 24 3. Do not meet criteria for dementia (consensus judgment of neuropsychologist and geriatrician)
Population-based study	1. Subjective memory complaint 2. Preserved intellectual functioning as estimated by performance on a vocabulary test 3. Memory impairment by detailed cognitive testing (no impairment on tests relating to other cognitive functions) 4. Intact activities of daily living 5. Absence of dementia
Population-based study	1. No dementia 2. Subjective memory complaint (self-reported) 3. Normal cognitive function (MMSE score higher than 1 SD below mean for age and education) 4. Objective memory impairment (1.5 SD below mean on Benton's Visula retention test) 5. Autonomy in activities of daily living (Katz activities of daily living scale)

The border zone between aging and dementia: cognitive and neuropathological changes

Age is the strongest risk factor for AD; the prevalence of AD doubles every 5 years after 65 years of age.[38] In spite of intense interest, the transition between normal aging and dementia remains difficult to delineate owing to indistinct cognitive and neuropathological boundaries. The wide variety of terms introduced to characterize aging-associated cognitive changes underscores the difficulty in distinguishing between aging and dementia (Table 1.4).

TABLE 1.4 Concepts of age-associated cognitive changes. The concept of mild cognitive impairment is one of many concepts that have attempted to characterize aging-associated cognitive changes. Adapted with permission from Ritchie *et al.* 2000.[19]

Concept	Criteria
Benign senescent forgetfulness[15]	Memory complaints, forgetful of remote events
Age-associated memory impairment[16]	Memory impairment on formal test at least 1 standard deviation below the norm for young adults
Aging-associated cognitive decline[17]	Impairment in memory or another cognitive domain greater than one standard deviation below norm for elderly
Aging-related cognitive decline[215]	Decline in cognitive functioning unrelated to specific mental or neurological problem
Mild cognitive decline[222]	Objectively measurable disorder of memory and learning secondary to systemic or cerebral disease or damage
Mild neurocognitive decline[215]	Same as mild cognitive decline with addition of perceptual-motor, linguistic, and executive deficits
Cognitive impairment no dementia[13]	Circumscribed memory impairment and low MMSE score, intact daily functioning
Mild cognitive impairment[20]	Memory complaint, objective cognitive deficit, and normal general and daily functioning

Aging and cognitive performance

A central but unresolved issue in defining prodromal dementia stages is determining which cognitive changes can be accepted as part of normal aging. Substantial individual differences exist in cognitive performance in non-demented individuals and those with early AD. As a result, the mildest cognitive changes ascribed to AD overlap considerably with cognitive performance in healthy aging individuals,[39–42] This has, in part, prompted the consideration that aging and AD are part of the same spectrum,[43] with cognitive decline and "senility" suggested to be an inevitable result of the aging process. There are, however, accumulating pathological and cognitive performance data from longitudinal studies to suggest that AD and aging may be distinct processes.

Although age differences have been consistently reported for some aspects of cognition,[44–46] methodological issues influence how these studies should be interpreted. Cross-sectional studies (i.e. data obtained from a group of individuals at a single time point) demonstrate performance deficits for older individuals when compared with younger persons. For instance, age differences are observed in measures of episodic memory, visuospatial ability, confrontation naming, and of psychomotor speed .[45–47] On the other hand, the magnitude of the deficits is generally small, and they do not appear to impair appreciably overall function or the ability to carry out activities of daily living.[48] These cross-sectional studies may be confounded by cohort effects related to generational differences in educational experiences, dietary and other environmental exposures, lifestyles, and other unknown factors. Moreover, cross-sectional samples may not be entirely normal. Because the incidence of AD increases dramatically with age, putatively "normal" samples of older individuals almost certainly include some with unrecognized incipient AD. This subset of individuals with undetected very mild impairment may exaggerate the cognitive decline that is attributed to age alone[49] (Figure 1.3).

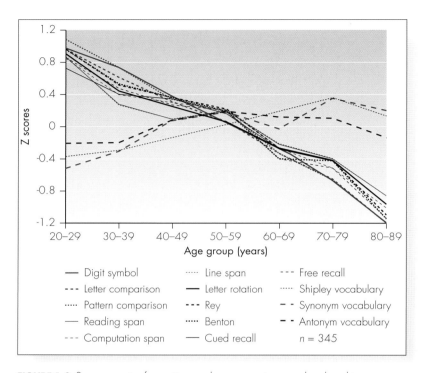

FIGURE 1.3 Some aspects of cognition, such as processing speed and working memory, are consistently reported to decline with age while others, such as vocabulary, remain stable. Methodological issues complicate these findings as longitudinal studies (following one individual over time) show less or no decline in cognition than cross-sectional studies (groups of individuals studied at one point in time). Reproduced from Dialogues in Clinical Neuroscience, with the permission of Les Laboratoires Servier, Neuilly-sur-Seine, France.

Evidence generated from longitudinal studies (i.e. following the same individuals prospectively over time) suggests AD is not inevitable with age. When strict criteria are employed to exclude even minimally demented individuals from longitudinal studies of the cognitively normal elderly, psychometric performance is shown to be surprisingly stable. Howieson et al.[50] evaluated 31 individuals with a mean age of 85 years at entry annually for up to 5 years. No cognitive declines were observed, even in domains predicted to demonstrate age effects, such as verbal memory. Rubin et al.[51] extended these findings by longitudinally studying 82 non-demented controls (mean age at entry, 72 years). Of these 82 non-demented controls, 60% remained non-demented up to 15 years later, with most showing no decline in annual psychometric performance on a standardized factor score (an indication of general cognitive performance). The large majority thus maintained stable cognitive performance with aging. In those individuals who eventually developed AD, the rate of change in psychometric performance before clinically detectable cognitive change occurred was generally not significantly different from those unaffected. Importantly, when subtle cognitive decline was clinically detected, an abrupt deterioration in psychometric performance was concurrently observed (Figures 1.4 and 1.5).

Storandt *et al.* replicated these findings in a larger cohort of individuals, including 230 carefully screened non-demented individuals followed

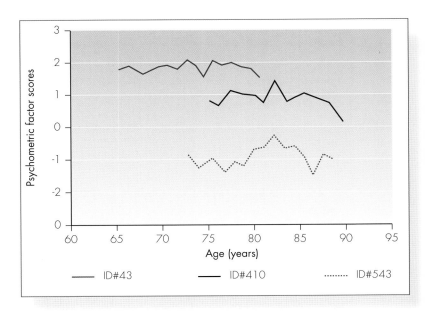

FIGURE 1.4 Demonstration of stable cognitive performance with age in 3 nondemented controls. Factor score is an index of general cognitive performance generated from a battery of neuropsychological tests. The large majority of a group of nondemented subjects followed for up to 15 years showed no decline in a standardized score of general cognitive performance.

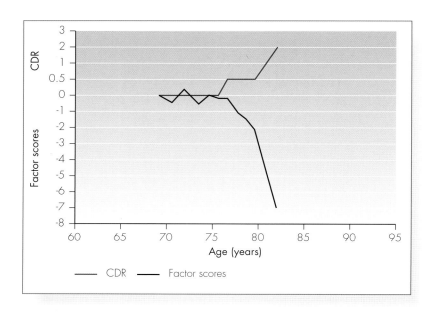

FIGURE 1.5 An abrupt decline in psychometric performance (green) occurs in this individual once subtle cognitive decline is detected (Clinical Dementia Rating (CDR) of 0.5, yellow). Stable cognitive performance is generally maintained up until the onset of a dementing illness, at which time a steep decline in performance occurs. Factor score is an index of cognitive performance. Reproduced with permission from Archives of Neurology, 1998, Vol 55: 395–401, © 1998, American Medical Association, all rights reserved.

for up to 20 years.[52] In this study, the "flat" trajectory of cognitive performance in healthy control subjects was again observed. None of the slope estimates for the non-demented individuals at any age was significantly different from zero. Those individuals with dementia ($n = 289$) showed rates of cognitive decline that increased with greater dementia severity. Those individuals with a diagnosis corresponding to MCI had significant declines in cognitive performance compared with controls (Figure 1.6).

Potential limitations of longitudinal studies include practice effects (i.e. repeated test administration may result in learning), ascertainment bias (healthy aging individuals may be more likely to volunteer), and selective attrition (more impaired subjects may drop out preferentially). While these limitations may offset declining

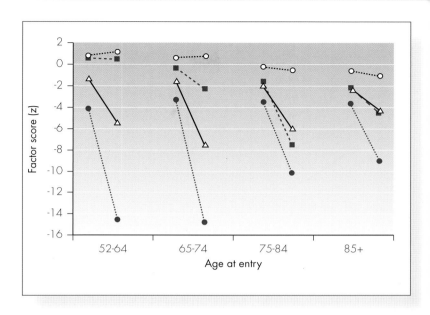

FIGURE 1.6 Cognitive change for age and dementia severity. The slopes represent the 10-year change in the general psychometric factor score (in SD units) as a function of age and dementia severity at entry. Non-demented controls (*open circles*) had a cognitive function trajectory which was not different from zero at any age. Individuals corresponding to MCI (*squares*, CDR 0.5 incipient dementia of the Alzheimer type (DAT)) demonstrated decline in cognition that was generally less severe than those at increased stages of dementia (*triangles* = CDR 0.5 DAT and filled circles = CDR 1). Only five individuals corresponding to MCI were present in the 52–64-years age group. Reproduced with permission from *The Neurologist 1995, 1: 326–344.*[22]

performances associated with age, the evidence nonetheless suggests that substantial cognitive decline need not be a part of truly healthy brain aging.[50,51,53–55]

AD and aging are unquestionably related. Careful assessment of elderly individuals over time shows that cognitively healthy elderly individuals maintain generally stable cognitive performance. At dementia onset, however, a steep decline in cognitive performance is observed, suggesting the onset of disease is distinct from the aging process. While subtle changes can be expected with age, cognitive decline interfering even mildly with the ability to perform daily functions is a marker of disease. Substantive cognitive decline should not be accepted as part of truly healthy aging. Conversely, even mild impairment may be an indicator of disease.

Neuropathology of Alzheimer's disease, non-demented aging and MCI

Histopathological features

The cardinal histopathological features of Alzheimer's disease (AD) are senile plaques and neurofibrillary tangles (NFT) in the cerebral cortex (Figure 2.1). The pathological diagnosis of AD rests on the presence of NFTs and amyloid plaques. Other pervasive microscopic changes include neuronal and synaptic loss, which are important in the pathogenesis and clinical manifestations of AD, but lack specificity and are less apparent with routine histopathological methods. Measures of synaptic or neuronal loss are not used in determining the pathological diagnosis.

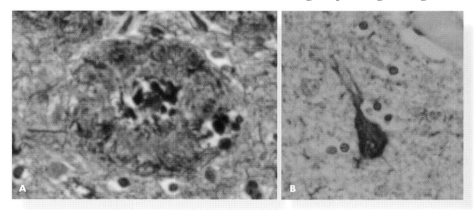

FIGURE 2.1 Plaques and neurofibrillary tangles are the pathological hallmarks of Alzheimer's disease. Plaques are composed primarily of extracellular accumulation of insoluble amyloid protein. Tangles are intracellular inclusions composed of aggregated tau proteins. Progressive aggregation of the abnormally phosphorylated tau protein is associated with the death of the neuron. **(A)** Neuritic amyloid plaque; Bielschovsky stain at 400x; **(B)** Neurofibrillary tangle; immunostaining for tau protein at 400x.

Plaques

The amyloid protein in AD is known as beta-amyloid peptide or Aβ. Aβ is revealed with the histopathological stains of congo-red, thioflavin S, and Bielschowsky silver stain, and with immunostaining.

An AD brain reveals large numbers of spherical, dense deposits in the cerebral cortex. Diffuse spherical plaques without a central core are commonly referred to as "senile plaques". Diffuse senile plaques may be among the earliest pathological changes of AD, later evolving into "neuritic" or "cored plaques", with a densely stained central core of abnormal, dystrophic neurites. Neuritic plaque density has been related to dementia severity, and thus may be more clinically relevant than the diffuse plaque.[56] Additionally, diffuse senile plaques are sometimes present in large numbers in older non-demented individuals and have been proposed to be a form of "pathological aging" (Figure 2.2).

Neurofibrillary pathology

Neurofibrillary degeneration is widespread in advanced AD. Neurofibrillary pathology takes several forms including NFTs, neuropil threads, and dystrophic neurites found in and around amyloid plaques. NFTs are argyrophilic fibrillar lesions in the neuronal perikarya and proximal dendrites and assume either "flame-shaped" or "globose" shapes. Neurofibrillary degeneration is visualized histopathologically using the Bielschowsky silver stain or Gallyas stain, among others. The major structural component of NFTs is the tau protein. Immunostaining for tau protein has been found to be the most sensitive method for detecting neurofibrillary pathology. Tau is a microtubule-associated protein that promotes the polymerization and stabilization of microtubules. The tau protein in NFTs is abnormally truncated, glycated, and phosphorylated. Phosphorylation of the protein affects its biological activity. While normal tau protein is able to dephosphorylate rapidly, abnormal tau protein contained in neurofibrillary tangles is resistant to dephosphorylation (Figures 2.3 and 2.4).

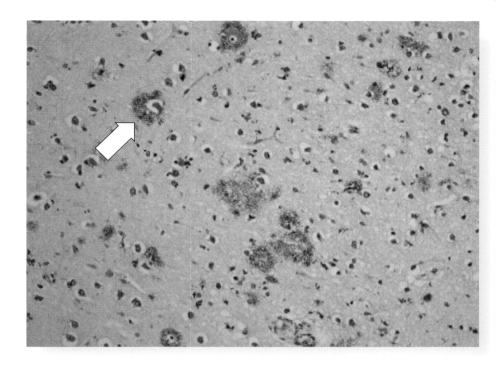

FIGURE 2.2 Frontal cortex from an 86-year-old woman with 12-year history of Alzheimer's disease revealing multiple amyloid plaques with silver Bielshovsky staining. At least one plaque shows a central neuritic core (*arrow*), while the majority are diffuse plaques.

Neuronal loss

Neuronal loss has been well documented throughout the AD-affected brain. Patients with even very mild AD have substantial loss of neuron number and volume in the entorhinal cortex and hippocampal CA1 region, areas highly vulnerable to the AD process.[57] Neuronal loss in the hippocampus may reach 57% compared to control brains with the CA1 region of the hippocampus most affected. Neuron

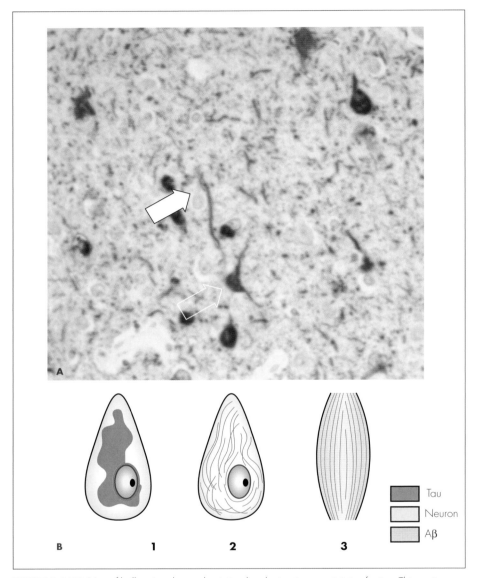

FIGURE 2.3 (A) Neurofibrillary tangles are best visualized using immunostaining for tau. This section reveals widespread, severe, neurofibrillary degeneration. Both flame-shaped (*open arrow*) and globose (*closed white arrow*) forms of neurofibrillary tangles are present. **(B)** Tau accumulates in neurons in a dispersed form **(1)** but eventually aggregates into paired helical filaments **(2)**. Death of the neuron eventually occurs with removal of cellular debris leaving only the extracellular ghost tangle **(3)**. Reproduced from Ellison and Love, Neuropathology 1998, with permission from Elsevier.[256]

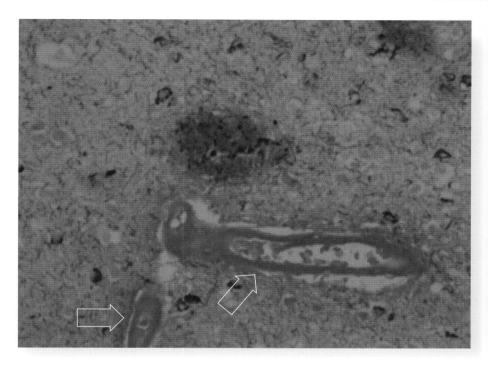

FIGURE 2.4 Neuritic changes commonly occur in amyloid plaques. These dual immunostains for both amyloid and tangle pathology reveal their co-occurrence. Using two different immunostains, amyloid is stained *red* and neurofibrillary changes (i.e. tau) *black*. Note blood vessels intensely stained with amyloid (amyloid angiopathy; denoted by *open arrows*).

loss in the hippocampus can be correlated significantly with the number of neurofibrillary tangles. The entorhinal cortex has marked neuron loss, reaching 90% in advanced AD; this correlates well with the earliest stages of cognitive decline. Cortical regions have been reported to have 50% neuron loss in AD, most prominent in upper cortical layers (lamina II and III), primarily involved in cortico–cortical connections. The mechanism of neuron loss is unclear, but has been postulated to involve direct or indirect consequence of Aβ deposition and may involve abnormal apoptosis (Figures 2.5 and 2.6).

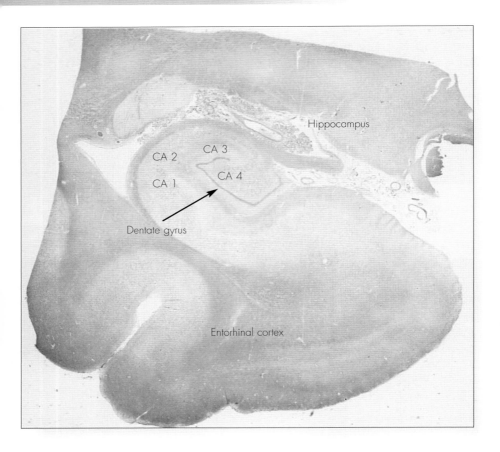

FIGURE 2.5 Photomicrograph of silver-stained section of a normal medial temporal lobe (coronal view). The hippocampus (particularly the CA1 region) and the entorhinal cortex have heavy plaque and tangle pathology burden in early AD and preclinical AD (individuals with pathological diagnosis of AD without clinical symptoms). Neuron loss in the entorhinal cortex is observable in the earliest forms of AD but not in preclinical AD. Thus, entorhinal cortical neuron loss may be important in expression of early AD clinical symptoms.

Topography of neuropathological changes

The progression of neurofibrillary tangle deposition in AD follows a hierarchical order, with involvement in a given area observed only if lower rank areas are affected. The entorhinal cortex is involved initially, followed later by the hippocampus and then regions of the

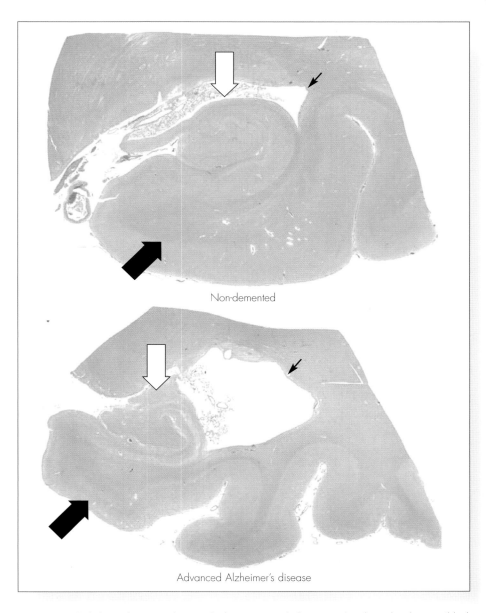

FIGURE 2.6 Pathological sections showing the hippocampus (*white arrows*) and entorhinal cortex (*black arrows*) in a non-demented individual (*left*) and an individual with late stage Alzheimer's disease (*right*). The temporal horn of the ventricle (*arrowhead*) is greatly enlarged in the demented individual due to severe atrophy of the entorhinal cortex and the hippocampus.

isocortex. This hierarchical progression of neurofibrillary degeneration is used in pathological staging of AD lesions. Interestingly, some degree of tangle deposition is present in all non-demented elderly adults. Tangle burden increases with age, and the deposition of NFTs in non-demented aging individuals follows the same hierarchical order as in AD, although tangle burden is less severe and is limited in distribution.

Aβ deposition is more diffuse and follows a less hierarchical pattern. The higher-order association areas are selectively vulnerable to Aβ deposition, while the primary sensory and motor neurons are largely spared. In contrast to NFT deposition, not all older non-demented adults have some degree of plaque deposition. Early in the course of AD, NFT and plaque deposition appear to be independent events. As the disease progresses, plaque deposition is associated with an increase in the number of tangles and the rate of tangle formation with age, suggesting an interaction between the two pathologies. Thus, the effect of amyloid deposition may be the acceleration of age-related tangle formation[58] (Figure 2.7).

Neuropathological AD diagnosis

In 1991, the Consortium to Establish a Registry for Alzheimer's Disease (CERAD) proposed standardized neuropathological criteria[59] for the post-mortem diagnosis of AD. The CERAD criteria are based on the semi-quantitative assessment of neuritic plaques in the frontal, temporal, and parietal neocortex. An age-related score is determined and integrated with clinical information regarding the presence or absence of dementia to yield the level of diagnostic certainty: definite, probable, or possible AD (Figure 2.8).

These, and other,[60,61] pathological criteria rest on two assumptions: (1) plaques in the neocortex increase as a function of age, and (2) plaques in AD are distinguished from aging only by their greater age-adjusted density. The basis of these assumptions comes from landmark studies demonstrating the presence of plaques and neurofibrillary tangles in the brains of older adults not considered demented during life.[62,63] These observations led to the idea that a

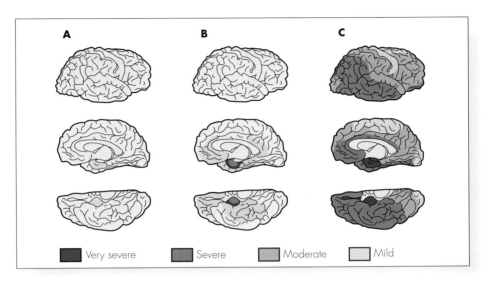

FIGURE 2.7 Neurofibrillary tangles accumulate in a predictable fashion with age and appear to be a ubiquitous accompaniment with aging. Accumulation of neurofibrillary tangles begins **(A)** in the medial temporal lobe (amygdala and entorhinal cortex), gradually extends into the **(B)** limbic system (hippocampus and cingulate cortices) and later throughout the entire isocortex **(C)**. The later stages of accumulation tend to be seen only in demented individuals, while tangle accumulation remains limited in extent in non-demented individuals. The presence of amyloid plaques appears to interact with tau pathology by increasing neurofibrillary tangle deposition. With permission, Ellison and Love, Neuropathology 1998.[256]

certain threshold of lesions must be reached before AD is clinically apparent.

It is particularly useful to examine closely the basis for these assumptions. Tomlinson and colleagues[63] evaluated the brains of 28 putatively non-demented patients with significant plaque pathology in 22 of the 28 patients. The findings led to the conclusion that there is no qualitative histological difference between aging and the dementia process: plaques are common to both and differ only in quantity.[64] This conclusion formed the basis for the development of subsequent histological criteria. Close examination of the non-demented control sample used by Tomlinson reveals that the data potentially are flawed. Tomlison and colleagues studied a group of elderly individuals with short life expectancies to increase the

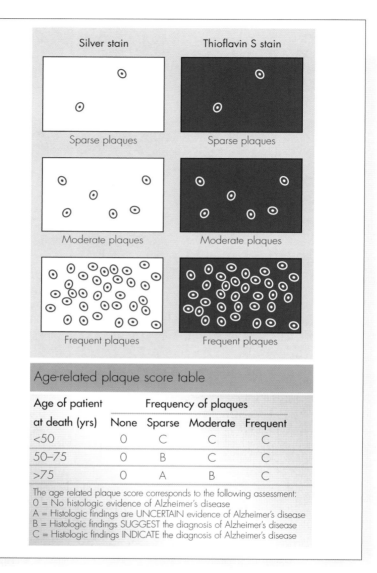

Age of patient	Frequency of plaques			
at death (yrs)	None	Sparse	Moderate	Frequent
<50	0	C	C	C
50–75	0	B	C	C
>75	0	A	B	C

The age related plaque score corresponds to the following assessment:
0 = No histologic evidence of Alzheimer's disease
A = Histologic findings are UNCERTAIN evidence of Alzheimer's disease
B = Histologic findings SUGGEST the diagnosis of Alzheimer's disease
C = Histologic findings INDICATE the diagnosis of Alzheimer's disease

FIGURE 2.8 CERAD neuropathological criteria[59] for the diagnosis of AD are based upon the semiquantitative assessment of plaque density. Observed cortical plaque densities are compared with the visual guide to determine severity of plaque burden: sparse, moderate or frequent. An age-related plaque score is determined through incorporating the age of the patient at death and the semiquantitative plaque burden. This score is then integrated with clinical information to yield the level of certainty of the diagnosis: definite, probable, or possible AD. Reproduced with permission from Neurology 1991, 41: 479–486.[59]

probability of neuropathological studies. The majority had been admitted in "terminal acute confusional states" to the geriatric unit of a general hospital or wards of a mental institution.[65] Although all were said to have "no positive evidence of a dementing illness", the authors conceded that the patients could not have been shown to have "cerebrated as well as they had done 20 years earlier". The threshold for "positive evidence" of dementia was notably higher than is prevalent today. Moreover, the "acute confusional states" are likely to have reflected a delirium, complicating mild underlying AD in at least some of the cases. The control sample therefore does not meet modern standards for non-demented aging.

Neuropathology of aging

The neuropathological boundary between aging and dementia remains controversial. In particular, there is uncertainty as to whether the classic pathological hallmarks of AD – senile plaques and NFTs – represent a disease-specific finding or can occur in normal brain aging. Accumulating evidence suggests that aging and AD are discrete processes, at least with regard to the appearance of senile plaques in the cerebral cortex.

Quantitative post-mortem studies indicate that slow neurofibrillary tangle accumulation occurs ubiquitously in non-demented adults[66], accumulating with age in a predictable pattern.[67] The distribution of NFTs generally remains limited to the medial temporal cortex.[68] This suggests that in a normal lifespan, the age-related accumulation of tangles may not result in dementia, although it may perhaps underlie cognitive complaints of "normal aging". In contrast, carefully assessed, non-demented control subjects up to 89 years of age have demonstrated little, if any, neocortical plaque pathology.[42,69] When neocortical plaque pathology is present, however, there appears to be an acceleration of the normal age-related NFT deposition and increased neocortical involvement.

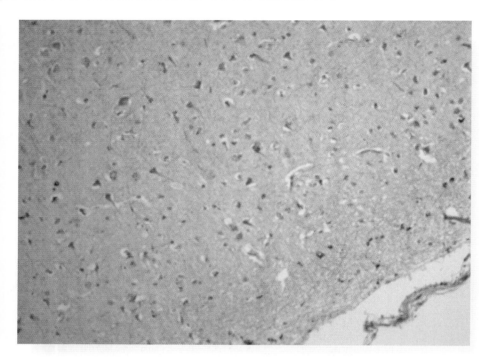

FIGURE 2.9 Frontal cortex from a 92-year-old woman with no cognitive decline (CDR 0); Bielshovsky stain. There are no amyloid plaques and neurofibrillary tangles present.

Regarding amyloid pathology, non-demented subjects appear to be separable into two groups based on amyloid plaque pathology: (1) little to no plaque pathology and (2) large numbers of diffuse senile plaques. In the first group, plaques can be entirely absent up to the ninth decade, indicating that healthy brain aging is possible (Figure 2.9). Some cognitively stable patients, however fall into the second group and have widely distributed neuritic and diffuse plaques throughout the neocortex and limbic areas. In terms of plaque density and distribution, these cognitively normal individuals resemble neuropathologically diagnosed AD. At least three potential explanations exist as to why these individuals are not demented: (1) they may not have AD, (2) they may have some protective factor that reduces the threshold of AD expression, or (3) the lesions have yet to culminate in substantial neuronal damage. If the latter is true, these subjects have a form of "preclinical" AD, defined as a stage when disease is present neuropathologically but has not yet produced clinically detectable cognitive changes (Figure 2.10).

Careful comparison of the brains from non-demented individuals, with and without AD pathology, fails to demonstrate differences in the number of neurons in the entorhinal cortex. Additionally, aging in non-demented controls between the sixth and ninth decades of life is not associated with loss of ERC neurons.[57] Thus, non-demented individuals, with and without "preclinical AD", do not appear to have important neuronal loss in the entorhinal cortex. In contrast,

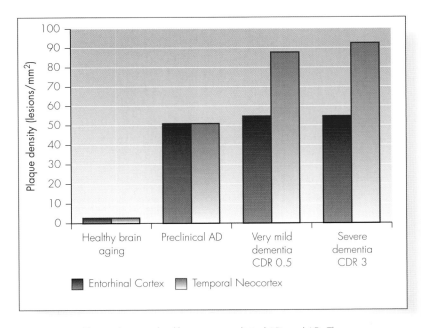

FIGURE 2.10 Plaque density in healthy aging, preclinical AD, and AD. The average density of plaques in the entorhinal cortex and temporal neocortex in non-demented, very mildly demented, and severely demented AD patients.[58] The CDR 0 group was divided into healthy brain aging (none to limited diffuse plaques) and preclinical AD (large numbers of neuritic and diffuse plaques). The preclinical AD cases resemble the CDR 0.5 cases pathologically, although lacking any cognitive impairment. Reprinted with permission of John Wiley & Sons, Inc.[58]

individuals in even the earliest stages of AD have significant senile plaques throughout the neocortex[42,70,71] and show a 32% reduction in entorhinal cortical neurons when compared with normal control values.[57] The occurrence of cell loss in these regions appears to be the event that sets apart the clinically recognizable cognitive changes of early AD from non-demented controls, including those with presumptive preclinical AD (Figure 2.11).

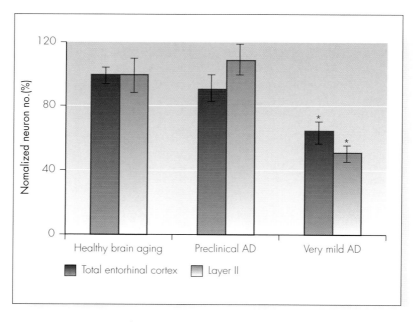

FIGURE 2.11 Neuron number in the entorhinal cortex in AD, preclinical AD, and healthy brain aging. The average number of neurons in the entorhinal cortex was similar in the healthy brain aging and preclinical AD groups.[249] Those with clinical symptoms of very mild AD have significantly fewer entorhinal cortical neurons. Reproduced with permission. Arch. Neurol, 2001; 58: 1395–1402, Copyright American Medical Association.[249]

These findings have led to a pathological model of dementia whereby neocortical plaques are the earliest pathological lesions of AD. Age-related deposition of neurofibrillary tangles is accelerated by the presence of amyloid plaques. Clinically recognizable cognitive decline becomes apparent with accumulation of substantial cell loss in the ERC and hippocampus cognitive changes of early AD (Table 2.1).

TABLE 2.1 Hypothetical clinicopathologic sequence in aging and AD.[249] Adapted with permission, Price et al. (2001).[249]

	Aging Normal	Preclinical AD AD	Very Mild AD AD
Pathological diagnosis			
Clinical Diagnosis	Normal (CDR 0)	Normal (CDR 0)	Very mild dementia (CDR 0.5)
Plaques (neocortex)	None, or few diffuse plaques	Many neuritic and diffuse plaques	Many neuritic and diffuse plaques
Tangles (entorhinal cortex and hippocampus/CA1)	+ to +++	+++	++++
Cell loss (entorhinal cortex)	None	Little to none	Substantial (30–60%)

Neuropathology of MCI

The neuropathological study of MCI individuals is essential to establish a causal link between the clinical symptoms and a neuropathological etiology. Several studies have shown that AD and MCI have remarkably similar neuropathological findings.[3–6,72,73] The neuropathological examination of individuals with very mild dementia and uncertain dementia corresponding to MCI overwhelmingly revealed pathological AD.[72] In an examination of brains from patients with MCI, AD, and normal controls, 61% of the MCI subjects had significant pathology to warrant a diagnosis of possible AD by CERAD criteria.[73] Pathological findings in the MCI and AD groups were virtually identical. Dramatic decreases in neuron number in layer II of the entorhinal cortex have been observed in subjects with MCI and AD with no apparent worsening of neuron loss in AD subjects compared with MCI subjects.[74] In another careful pathological study, individuals with MCI had increased neuritic plaques and neurofibrillary tangles compared to normal controls. Neuritic plaques were not different in MCI versus AD although there appeared to be a gradient of increasing neurofibrillary tangle pathology from normal controls, MCI, and AD participants.[3] These studies, taken together, suggest the neuropathology of MCI overwhelmingly is that of AD.

Does a subset of MCI patients actually have early Alzheimer's disease?

In the broadest sense of the term, MCI is a heterogeneous condition with a lengthy differential diagnosis. Many individuals diagnosed with MCI progress to further stages of cognitive impairment and clearly develop the manifestations of AD. On the other hand, not all MCI patients will progress, and some may even improve. Longitudinal studies showing that a significant proportion of MCI individuals will progress to AD suggest that at least some individuals are likely to be in the earliest stages of AD. Thus, the major diagnostic challenge lies in identifying more uniformly those individuals with early AD-related cognitive changes rather than a group with heterogeneous etiologies.

Clinical studies

Clinical studies of MCI subjects demonstrate patterns of cognitive deficits and clinical features that are similar to AD, only less severe.[20,37] Genetic risk factors (i.e. *ApoE*) are similar in AD and MCI patients.[76] Individuals with MCI and AD share similar neuropsychiatric profiles. Neuropsychiatric symptoms such as agitation, depression, apathy, delusions, hallucinations and sleep impairment are common to AD, affecting up to 80% of individuals with dementia over the course of the disease. Lyketsos *et al.*[77] assessed neuropsychiatric symptoms in both MCI and AD patients; they found their prevalence in MCI subjects to be intermediate to that of AD and normal controls. Neuropsychiatric symptoms were exhibited by 43% of the MCI subjects compared with 75% of the dementia subjects, with depression and apathy being most common in both groups.

Neuroimaging

Structural and functional imaging techniques have been used in the assessment of MCI patients.[78–80] CT (computed tomography) and MRI (magnetic resonance imaging) studies have primarily assessed the morphology of the hippocampus, while functional techniques such as single-photon emission computed tomography (SPECT), positron emission tomography (PET), and magnetic resonance spectroscopy (MRS) have focused primarily on patterns of metabolic deficits. The general consensus from these studies is that MCI and AD share many neuroimaging features in common.[81]

Medial temporal lobe volume loss has been reported in both AD[82–84] and MCI[85] subjects compared with non-demented controls, with the degree of volume loss greater in the AD subjects. Substantial evidence exists that MRI volumetrics are a valid biomarker for AD pathological progression, indirectly detecting cell loss and correlating with AD neuropathological burden.[86–88] In a longitudinal study of MCI subjects, hippocampal atrophy at baseline predicted subsequent conversion to AD. Individuals with very mild AD (CDR 0.5) have been shown to have significantly reduced bilateral hippocampal volumes when compared with healthy controls.[89] Thus, both MCI subjects and those in the earliest stages of AD have similar anatomic involvement of the medial temporal lobes (Figure 2.12).

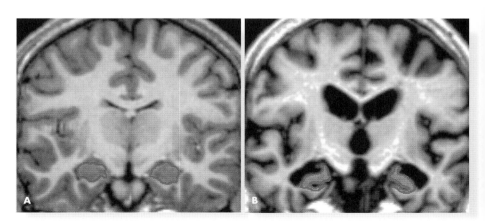

FIGURE 2.12 The hippocampi of a young male and an 86 year old woman with Alzheimer disese are outlined in coronal section (red). The hippocampi of the older individual are substantially atrophied as demonstrated by the size and the prominence of the temporal ventricular horns. (Courtesy of Denise Head and Randy L. Buckner)

Functional imaging studies using SPECT and PET suggest similar distribution of metabolic defects in AD and MCI subjects. AD-associated hypometabolism in posterior cortical regions has been reported consistently and is a proposed early diagnostic marker of AD.[90,91] MCI subjects have demonstrated posterior cortical hypoperfusion intermediate between that found in normal controls and in patients with AD.[92] Questionable AD patients who later converted to AD had reduced perfusion of posterior cortical regions and the hippocampus, an area involved early in the neuropathological AD process, when compared with those who did not decline.[93]

The considerable overlap in clinical and neuroimaging characteristics suggests that a subset of individuals identified with the MCI criteria in fact may have the earliest cognitive changes of AD. It has been argued that a dichotomous distinction of MCI from dementia and the assessment of "conversion" to dementia limits our ability to capture the heterogeneous outcomes of this patient group,[28] raising the question of whether a dichotomous distinction of MCI from AD is appropriate. Thus, more uniformly identifying those individuals with early AD-related cognitive changes, rather than a group with heterogeneous etiologies, remains the major diagnostic challenge.

Detecting and diagnosing MCI and early AD

"The best diagnostic test is a careful history and physical and mental status examination by a physician with a knowledge of and interest in dementia and the dementing diseases. Such an evaluation is time consuming, but nothing can replace it."

NIH Consensus Statement, 1987[94]

Early detection

An estimated 20 million individuals worldwide are afflicted with Alzheimer's disease (AD), of which 4 million are in the U.S.A. Incident cases of AD are expected to nearly triple in the U.S.A. over the next 50 years.[95] Unfortunately, these figures are likely under-estimates given dementia's common under-recognition.[96] Currently, the majority of AD diagnoses are made when dementia is readily apparent. A median of 1.6 years elapses between family recognition and consultation. Diagnosis occurs on average about 3.5–5.5 years after the first symptoms.[97] These figures indicate that AD is widely under-diagnosed and under-treated.

The primary physician is in an important position to detect the earliest cognitive changes of dementia. This is not always an easy task. The widespread myth that aging inevitably brings forgetfulness has profound effects on the views of both lay people and physicians, hindering the early recognition and diagnosis of cognitive decline. Moreover, the insidious nature of dementing illnesses and the presence of co-morbid conditions blurs the meaning of decline from prior levels of function.

It is not uncommon to reserve the diagnosis of AD for moderate to severe cases, reflecting uncertainty in distinguishing mild dementia from normal aging. In the moderate to severe dementia stage, functional status is severely disrupted and the pathological lesions of neuronal loss, amyloid plaques, and neurofibrillary tangles are firmly established.

The advent of approved drugs for the treatment of AD has led to a growing interest in the early diagnosis of the disease. The recognition and diagnosis of AD in its earliest stages is important for investigating proposed etiologic mechanisms, putative biomarkers, and potential disease-altering therapies. Moreover, many patients and families have an interest in the cause of cognitive changes, and early diagnosis can relieve anxiety stemming from this diagnostic uncertainty. Patients are also able to play an active role in planning and preparing for the future before they are no longer capable.

Recognition of MCI and early AD

The key information needed to diagnose dementia and create a differential diagnosis comes primarily from clinical information. Clinically diagnosing AD rests on determining whether cognitive decline is present to such a degree as to interfere with function in usual activities. The 2001 American Academy of Neurology (AAN) practice parameter on the diagnosis of dementia recommended routine use of the criteria elaborated in the Diagnostic and Statistical Manual (DSM).[98] The criteria's key principles include (1) cognitive decline and (2) interference with functioning as the ultimate validation of the presence of dementia (Table 3.1).

TABLE 3.1 Definition of dementia: DSM IV[215]

- Impairment in short- and long-term memory, associated with impairment in abstract thinking, impaired judgment, other disturbances of higher cortical function, or personality change
- The disturbance is severe enough to interfere significantly with work or usual social activities or relationships with others

Determining whether these criteria are met involves the following: (1) assessing the presenting problem; (2) obtaining information from someone who knows the patient well, such as a family member (i.e. obtaining an informant-based history); (3) conducting physical and neurological examinations; and (4) evaluating the cognitive, behavioral, and functional status of the patient. Dementia remains a clinical diagnosis, and no test replaces an assessment by an experienced physician (Table 3.2).

TABLE 3.2 Clinical hallmarks of dementia

- Gradual onset
- Progressive decline
- Memory loss
- Other cognitive domains impaired
- Interferes with function

The diagnosis of AD, by far the most common form of dementia in the U.S.A., has been standardized with criteria developed by the Work Group of the National Institute of Neurologic and Communicative Disorders and Stroke and the Alzheimer's Disease and Associated Disorders Association (NINCDS–ADRDA). The NINCDS–ADRDA criteria[99] established three levels of confidence for the diagnosis of AD: probable, possible, and definite (Table 3.3). Definite Alzheimer's disease can be diagnosed only by autopsy. Probable AD is diagnosed "if there is a typical insidious onset of dementia with progression, and if there are no other systemic or brain diseases that could account for the progressive memory and other cognitive deficits". Possible AD is diagnosed when there are variations in the presentation or course of dementia, such as early or disproportionate language disturbance, or when another potentially dementing disorder (e.g. stroke) is present but is not believed to be responsible for dementia.

The application of the NINCDS–ADRDA criteria shows good sensitivity (81%) and reasonable specificity (70%).[98] When applied

TABLE 3.3 Alzheimer's disease: NINCDS – ADRDA criteria[99]

1. Probable AD:
   a. Measurable deficits in two or more areas of cognition
   b. No disturbance in consciousness
   c. Progressive worsening
   d. Onset between 40 and 90
   e. Absence of systemic disease or other brain disease that could account for the deficits
   f. Diagnostic support:
      i. Progressive deterioration
      ii. Impaired ADLs
      iii. Family history of similar disorder
      iv. Normal LP/EEG
      v. Atrophy on CT
   g. Other consistent clinical features include plateaus in the course of progression, associated symptoms of depression, insomnia, incontinence, delusions, illusions, sexual disorders, seizures (in advanced disease); neurological abnormalities such as increased tone, myoclonus, gait disorders
   h. Features making diagnosis unlikely include sudden onset; focal neuro signs; seizures or gait disturbance early in course

2. Possible AD:
   a. Dementia syndrome with variations in onset, course or presentation or the presence of other problems or disorders that may produce dementia but are not considered the cause of dementia

3. Definite AD:
   a. Clinical criteria met
   b. Histopathologic evidence present at autopsy

by dementia experts, these criteria yield a diagnostic accuracy of 85–95%, as validated by neuropathological examination. The development of standard, reliable, and valid clinical diagnostic criteria and staging methods has led to improvements in diagnostic accuracy; these improvements allow meaningful comparison of therapeutic trial results and the detection of AD at earlier stages in its development. The concept of MCI is a direct result of these advances.

Informant-based history

Because each individual's usual activities vary according to native intelligence and their educational and occupational experiences, the history of a meaningful decline must be individualized. This means gaining information about cognitive changes from someone who knows the patient well, such as the spouse or a family member. The memory loss of MCI and early AD is generally well compensated. Individuals perform independently in the community, and their symptoms are not readily apparent to those of casual contact. Observations from an attentive family member, relative, or friend describing cognitive changes interfering even mildly with the patient's usual function are essential in making a confident diagnosis. Family members may be inclined to disregard cognitive changes; however, careful probing of the informant often reveals that the individuals are not performing at their prior level. The perceptions of a knowledgeable informant have been shown to be sensitive and reliable for detecting early dementia.[32–36]

Additionally, self-reported memory complaints correlate poorly with actual cognitive performance and do not predict development of dementia.[101,102] Memory complaints in "worried-well" individuals tend to be associated more with personality traits and depression rather than with dementia,[101] and self-reported memory complaints not corroborated by an informant's testimony of cognitive decline can be an important clue. However, these self-reported complaints should not necessarily be dismissed as benign, as patients with early AD often retain some insight into their difficulties. On the other hand, self-reports claiming an absence of problems should not be taken at face value, and careful probing of an informant is important and often essential to revealing the cognitive changes of dementia.

Common examples of early AD-related cognitive changes include a decline in the ability to manage the checkbook or household finances, difficulty with driving (e.g. getting lost or disoriented, and indecisiveness), decline in cooking skills (e.g. from poor planning and organizational skills), difficulty using household appliances (e.g.

microwave oven, remote control, or telephone), and impaired performance of hobbies (e.g. cards, reading, or golf). Importantly, a subject need not relinquish activities fully to meet the interference criterion but must simply perform them less well than before owing to cognitive loss (Table 3.4).

TABLE 3.4 Common symptoms of MCI and early AD

Memory loss
- Forgetful of pertinent details of recent events
- Repeating questions
- Misplacement of items

Executive dysfunction
- Difficulties managing checkbook/household finances
- Decline in cooking skills
- Decline in home repair/maintenance skills
- Trouble operating household appliances
  - Microwave, remote control, telephone

Daily Activities
- Impaired performance in hobbies
  - Playing cards
  - Reading
- Difficulty driving
  - Getting lost
  - Indecisiveness
  - Minor or major accidents
- Shopping
  - Frequent trips for forgotten items
  - Doubling up on items

Unfortunately, when the informant is not observant or is unavailable (or, in today's practices, there is insufficient time for a physician to interview the informant in addition to seeing the patient), true decline can be difficult to identify. In these cases, impaired performance can be inferred from the patient only when a basic activity (e.g. dressing or bathing) is all but relinquished. Another difficulty is in separating the impact of co-morbid conditions on an individual's daily functioning from the effect of cognitive decline. The presence of medical illnesses and physical ailments can lead to significant changes in activity, confounding the determination, by physician and family alike, of a change from a previous level of functioning. These challenges make the diagnosis of early dementia more difficult.

We have found that, in a matter of minutes, the collateral source can be probed for the presence of key features suggestive of early AD. These include repetition of questions and statements, judgment problems, difficulty using a tool or appliance, difficulty remembering appointments, and consistent problems with thinking and memory.

Neurological examination

In mild and even moderate AD, focal neurological abnormalities are infrequent. The neurological examination is performed primarily to evaluate for the presence of any signs suggestive of another dementing illness. The neurological examination should therefore be focused on evaluating for the presence of focal upper motor neuron signs, extrapyramidal signs, and prominent aphasia and apraxia (Table 3.5).

TABLE 3.5 Features suggestive of other dementing illness

Parkinsonism → dementia with Lewy bodies, corticobasal degeneration

Language
    Naming impairment → progressive non-fluent aphasia
    Comprehension impairment → semantic aphasia

Apraxia → corticobasal degeneration
Myoclonus → prion disease (Creutzfeldt-Jakob disease)

Mild impairments in language and praxis are commonly encountered in AD, although memory loss remains the prominent symptom. Language impairments often begin with mild word-finding difficulties, manifested as circumlocutions (substituting the desired word with a description or series of shorter words) and halting speech. Unexplained language impairments with relative sparing of memory may indicate the presence of a variant of frontotemporal lobar degeneration such as non-fluent progressive aphasia or semantic dementia.

Apraxia, a disorder of skilled movement despite intact strength, sensation, and coordination, will develop as the typical AD progresses, but it is not a prominent, early manifestation. Apraxia in mild AD patients is commonly characterized as substitution of the individual's hand as object, for instance using their fist to represent a hammer rather than grasping an imaginary hammer. Severe apraxia, often unilateral, may indicate corticobasal degeneration.

Focal neurological deficits such as mild hemiparesis, unilateral visual field deficit, or Babinski sign may indicate the presence of significant vascular disease, which commonly coexists with AD, and may play a role in the symptomatic expression of AD.[103]

The presence of increased tone and a Parkinsonian gait early in the course may indicate dementia with Lewy bodies or Parkinson's dementia. Extrapyramidal signs are common in advanced AD but are generally not prominent early in the course. Prominent unilateral extrapyramidal signs may indicate corticobasal degeneration. Prominent myoclonus may indicate Creutzfeldt-Jakob disease, particularly if accompanying a rapidly progressive dementing illness, although myoclonus can also be encountered in AD (Table 3.5).

Laboratory and radiological evaluation

Structural neuroimaging is recommended in the form of either magnetic resonance imaging (MRI) or non-contrast computed tomography (CT). The basis of this recommendation is evidence that up to 5% of patients with dementia have a clinically significant structural lesion that would not have been predicted based on the history or examination.[104] These potential lesions include brain neoplasms, subdural hematomas, or normal-pressure hydrocephalus. However, fully reversible dementia due to unsuspected causes is rare. The AAN practice parameter reported insufficient evidence to recommend single-photon emission computed tomography (SPECT) or positron emission tomography (PET) in the routine evaluation of dementia patients. Additionally, PET and SPECT imaging have not been shown to be cost-effective for dementia diagnosis.[105]

Depression, B12 deficiency, and hypothyroidism are common co-morbidities in patients with suspected dementia, and screening for these treatable disorders is recommended (Table 3.6).[98] Depression coexists with AD in up to 12% of demented patients,[106] and a few reports have attributed dementia to B12 deficiency and hypothyroidism.[107] In most individuals, treatment of these disorders is unlikely to reverse completely cognitive deficits, and cognitive improvements in demented patients given B12 and thyroid replacement are questionable.[98] Nevertheless, the high frequency of these co-morbidities and the potential for amelioration of cognitive symptoms necessitates screening. Routine screening for syphilis is no longer recommended unless syphilis risk factors exist or there is evidence of infection ; this represents a change from the 1994 practice parameter.[108]

TABLE 3.6 Basic laboratory assessment for cognitive impairment

Neuroimaging
- CT or MRI

Laboratory
- Thyroid
- Vitamin B12
- Syphilis (only if clinically indicated)

Psychometric/mental status testing

Mental status tests should be used primarily to confirm the presence of cognitive deficits and not as a method of diagnosis. Mental status tests cannot, certainly at the initial evaluation, indicate whether the individual has declined from previous levels of cognitive abilities or determine the presence of impairment sufficient to interfere with accustomed activities. This information must be collected from the informant interview. Testing is useful in demonstrating a pattern of deficits consistent with an AD pattern (primary deficits in memory and executive function) and to monitor dementia progression over time through serial testing. Over-reliance on cognitive test performance, in addition to failure to incorporate an informant's observations about an individual's cognitive function in relation to past abilities, results in the under-recognition of mild AD.

The determination of normal and abnormal performance on psychometric tests uses arbitrary cut-off points and standard deviations for a group mean of memory performance. These means are not always applicable to an individual. Cognitive tests, such as the mini-mental state examination (MMSE)[109] are influenced by age, education,[110] race,[111] and gender and show large measurement error. These factors often make cognitive tests insensitive to early-stage AD.[39–41] The performance of non-demented aging and very mild and mild AD individuals on widely used cognitive scales such as the MMSE and the Blessed Scale-cognitive portion[65] show considerable overlap between the groups (Table 3.7). This suggests that over-reliance on neuropsychological tests would exclude some individuals experiencing interference with their usual functions who are still performing within the arbitrary range of normal.

In 2001, the American Academy of Neurology conducted an evidenced-based review of the diagnosis of MCI.[112] The report found that general cognitive screening instruments are useful in the detection of dementia in those individuals with suspected cognitive decline (i.e. MCI). Owing to their insensitivity in detecting dementia, however, they are not recommended as a general screen of

TABLE 3.7 Selected cognitive instruments used in detection of dementia.[112] Multiple cognitive assessment tools have been used in the detection of dementia. The most widely used screening tool, the MMSE, has been shown to be insensitive. The seven-minute screen is sensitive and specific in detecting dementia in a highly selected sample but is unlikely to retain this capacity in day-to-day practice. Moreover, it has not been assessed in early AD individuals. We recently showed the clock-drawing test to be insensitive in detecting early AD.[117] Table adapted with permission from Petersen et al. (2001).[112]

Instrument (cutoff)	Sensitivity	Specificity
MMSE (score < 24)[114]	63%	96%
MMSE (bottom 10%)[113]	49%	92%
MMSE (decline of 4 points/1–4 years)[250]	82%	99%
Seven-minute screen[118]	92%	96%
Clock-drawing test[116]	85%	85%
CDR[251]	92%	94%
IQCODE[252]	89%	88%

asymptomatic individuals. Given an MCI patient's increased risk of developing overt dementia, the AAN concluded that clinical evaluation and follow-up monitoring of MCI individuals using psychometric tools was justified.

Psychometric tools include commonly used cognitive screening tools (i.e. the MMSE, the seven-minute screen, and the clock-drawing test), neuropsychological batteries (i.e. Mattis Dementia Rating Scale), and informant-based instruments [including CDR, GDS, and informant questionnaire on cognitive decline in the elderly (IQCODE)].

Dementia-screening instruments

Mini-mental state examination

The mini-mental state examination (MMSE)[109] is a widely used screening tool for cognitive dysfunction that briefly assesses orientation, memory, language, and visuospatial skills on a 30-point scale. Many MCI studies use an MMSE score greater than 24 to define intact general cognitive functioning as part of the MCI criteria.

Despite its widespread use, the MMSE has limited use in discriminating between demented and non-demented patients, particularly when used in isolation.[112] In a population-based study, the MMSE was found to be only 49% sensitive in detecting dementia as defined by a CDR of $\geq$ 0.5.[113] Another study indicated that the standard cutoff score of < 24 was insensitive (63%) in detecting dementia at 1-year follow-up in individuals with cognitive complaints.[114] The MMSE is more useful when it is used to longitudinally monitor cognitive performance. For instance, in a longitudinal study of 3,513 elderly subjects, a decline of 4 points over 1–4 years was 82% sensitive in detecting dementia. The positive predictive value of the test, however, is dependent on the population sampled. When administered to a population with a high prevalence of dementia (20%) the positive predictive value is 91%, while in a population with a low prevalence (5%), the positive predictive value is only 68%. The population assessed thus has a significant impact on the usefulness of the test. Thus, the MMSE has limited usefulness in discriminating demented and non-demented individuals in the general population (Table 3.8).

Clock-drawing test

The clock-drawing test[115] has become popular as a screening instrument for AD. The test taps into a broad range of cognitive domains that may be impaired in AD, such as memory, spatial knowledge, abstract thinking, planning, concentration, and visuoconstructive skills. A review of published studies reported a mean sensitivity of 85% in the ability of the clock test to differentiate those individuals with probable AD from normal individuals.[116] We studied the usefulness of the clock-drawing test as a screen for very mild dementia (CDR 0.5).[117] Our results indicate that the test is useful in detecting mild dementia (CDR 1) but that its ability to detect the earliest forms of dementia was poor; in addition, those with very mild dementia did not differ significantly from cognitively normal older adults (Figure 3.1).

TABLE 3.8 Mini-mental state exam

"Now I would like to ask you some questions to check your memory and concentration. Some of them may be easy and some of them may be hard"

Error	Correct	1
0	1	1. What is the YEAR? _____
0	1	2. What is the SEASON of the year? _____
0	1	3. What is the DATE? _____
0	1	4. What is the DAY OF THE WEEK? _____
0	1	5. What is the MONTH?" _____
0	1	6. Can you tell me where we are? _____ (What STATE are we in?)
0	1	7. What country are we in? _____ (What MAJOR RIVER are we near?)
0	1	8. What CITY/TOWN are we in? _____
0	1	9. What FLOOR of the building are we on? _____
0	1	10. What is the NAME or ADRESS of this place? _____

11. I am going to name three objects. After I've said them, I want you to repeat them. Remember what they are because I am going to ask you to name them again in a few minutes. Please repeat the names for me.

Error	Correct	
0	1	*APPLE* _____
0	1	*TABLE* _____ (Score first try. Repeat objects for three trials only)
0	1	*PENNY* _____

12. Now I am going to give you a word and ask you to spell it forwards and backwards. The word is *WORLD*. First, can you spell it forwards? (OK Help) Now spell it backwards. (Repeat if necessary and help subject spell the word forward, if necessary.)

Error	Correct	
0	1	D _____
0	1	L _____
0	1	R _____ _____ Score number of letters given in correct order.
0	1	O _____
0	1	W _____

Error	Correct	
0	1	13. *APPLE* _____
0	1	14. *TABLE* _____ "What were the three objects I asked you to remember?"
0	1	15. *PENNY* _____

Error	Correct	
0	1	16. (Show *WRIST WATCH*) What is this called? _____
0	1	17. (Show *PENCIL*) What is this called? _____
0	1	18. I would like you to repeat a phrase after me: *NO IF'S, AND'S OR BUTS* (only 1 trial)
0	1	19. Read the words on this page and then do what it says: CLOSE YOUR EYES (Code correct if subject closes eyes.)

20. I am going to give you a piece of paper. When I do, take the paper in your right hand, fold the paper in half with both hands, and put the paper down on your lap.

Error	Correct	
0	1	*RIGHT HAND* _____
0	1	*FOLDS IN 1/2* _____ (Read full statement, then hand over paper.
0	1	*PLACE IN LAP* _____ Do not repeat instructions or coach.)
0	1	21. Write any complete SENTENCE on that piece of paper for me. (+ ____
0	1	22. Here is a DRAWING. Please copy the drawing on the same paper. − ____) (Score correct if the two five-sided figures intersect to form a four sided figure and if all angles in the five-sided figures are preserved.)

_____ **TOTAL SCORE** (The sum of the score for all 22 questions): **MINI MENTAL STATE EXAM**

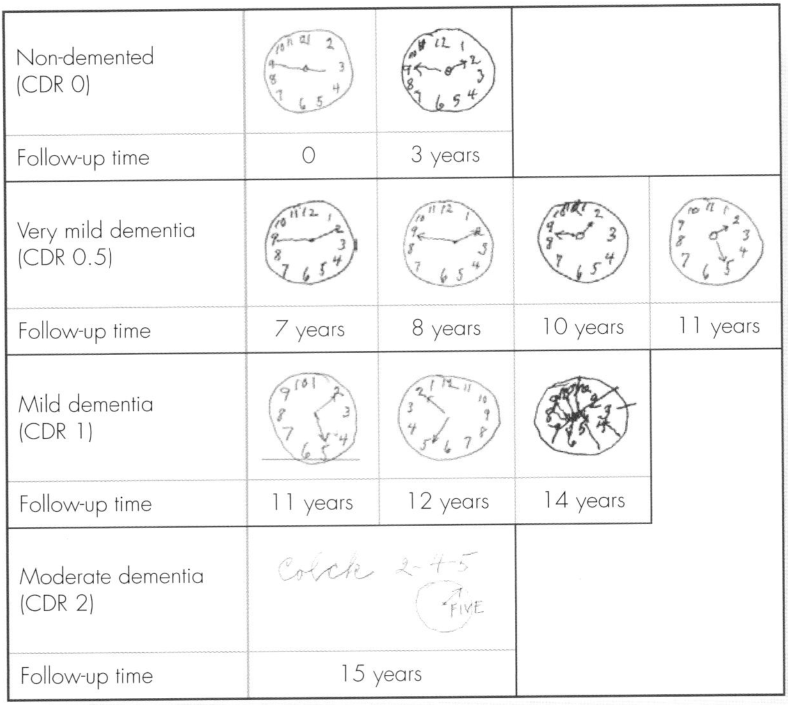

Non-demented (CDR 0)			
Follow-up time	0	3 years	
Very mild dementia (CDR 0.5)			
Follow-up time	7 years	8 years	10 years	11 years
Mild dementia (CDR 1)			
Follow-up time	11 years	12 years	14 years
Moderate dementia (CDR 2)			
Follow-up time	15 years		

FIGURE 3.1 A selection of annual clock drawings from an individual followed longitudinally over 15 years. The subject was asked to "Draw a clock with all the numbers; then show me 2:45". Symptomatic onset of Alzheimer's disease was recognized at 7 years when the patient was given a CDR 0.5 rating. The first incorrect clock was drawn at 11 years, 4 years after onset of symptomatic AD when the subject placed the hands on the clock incorrectly (2:25 rather than 2:45). Clock drawing is insensitive to detecting very early dementia, limiting its utility as a screening tool.

Seven-minute screen

The 7-min screening instrument is comprised of enhanced cued recall, category fluency, Benton Temporal Orientation Test, and the clock-drawing test.[118] The test was administered to 60 consecutive patients diagnosed clinically with AD referred to memory-disorder clinics and 60 age-matched controls recruited through advertising. The sensitivity in discriminating these highly selected AD patients from normal controls was 92%, and the specificity was 96%. It is likely that the sensitivity and specificity of the test would be reduced in day-to-day practice due to the referral-based sample.[118] Moreover, the test has not been assessed in a sample of early-stage AD.

Dementia staging instruments

CDR

The clinical dementia rating (CDR)[119,120] is a dementia staging instrument used to rate cognitive function in six domains: memory, orientation, judgment and problem solving, community affairs, home and hobbies , and personal care. These domains are rated along five levels of impairment from none to maximal (rated as 0, 0.5, 1, 2, and 3) using a structured interview of the patient and a knowledgeable informant. Only impairment caused by cognitive dysfunction is rated. Community affairs and home and hobbies assess instrumental activities of daily living and vary according to the individual's accustomed activities. Examples include job performance, skills in driving, home repairs, household finances, shopping, cooking, and card games. Personal care represents basic activities of daily living such as dressing, bathing, grooming, eating, and continence (Table 3.9).

A global CDR is determined from the individual ratings in each domain (or "box scores"), using a set of scoring rules. Not all domains need to be rated the same. CDR 0 indicates no dementia, while CDR 0.5 represents very mild, CDR 1 mild, CDR 2 moderate, and CDR 3 severe dementia. The CDR 0.5-stage originally was designated "questionable dementia", but we have recognized that this stage often represents the earliest symptomatic stage of AD; it has subsequently been re-designated as "very mild dementia".

The CDR has been shown to have high inter-rater reliability (for physicians[121] and non-physicians[122]) and is independent from psychometric test scores. A more quantitative version of the scale can be used through summing the ratings in each of the six categories ("sum of boxes"), and the six categories are directly linked to validated diagnostic criteria in AD.[123] These features make the CDR a useful, clinically based dementia-staging tool.

TABLE 3.9 Clinical dementia rating (CDR)

	None 0	Questionable 0.5
Memory	No memory loss or slight inconsistent forgetfulness	Consistent slight forgetfulness; partial recollection of events; "benign" forgetfulness
Orientation	Fully oriented	Fully oriented except for slight difficulty with time relationships
Judgment and problem solving	Solves everyday problems and handles business and financial affairs well; judgment good in relation to past performance	Slight impairment in solving problems, similarities, and differences
Community affairs	Independent function at usual level in job, shopping, volunteer and social groups	Slight impairment in these activities
Home and hobbies	Life at home, hobbies, and intellectual interests well maintained	Life at home, hobbies, and intellectual interests slightly impaired
Personal care	Fully capable of self-care	

Score only as decline from previous usual level due to cognitive loss, not impairment due to other factors.

Global deterioration scale

The global deterioration scale (GDS)[124] is a dementia-staging instrument with seven stages representing different levels of impairment. Stage 1 represents no cognitive impairment. Stages 2 and 3 correlate best with MCI and are considered the pre-dementia stages. Stages 4 to 7 are considered the stages of dementia. Beginning in stage 5, the individual can no longer survive without assistance. Stage 7 represents the most severe cognitive impairment. The levels are based on empiric observations of typical symptoms and behavior clusters (Table 3.10).

Mild 1	Moderate 2	Severe 3
Moderate memory loss; more marked for recent events; defect interferes with everyday activities "benign"	Severe memory loss; only highly learned material retained; new material rapidly lost	Severe memory loss; only fragments remain recollection of events;
Moderate difficulty with time relationships; oriented for place at examination; may have geographic disorientation elsewhere	Severe difficulty with time relationships; usually disoriented to time, often to place	Oriented to person only
Moderate difficulty in handling problems, similarities, and differences; social judgment usually maintained	Severely impaired in handling problems, similarities, and differences; social judgment usually impaired	Unable to make judgments or solve problems
Unable to function independently at these activities although may still be engaged in some; appears normal to casual inspection	No pretense of independent function outside home Appears well enough to be taken to functions outside a family home	Appears too ill to be taken to functions outside a family home
Mild but definite impairment of function at home; more difficult chores abandoned; more complicated hobbies and interests abandoned	Only simple chores preserved; very restricted interests, poorly maintained	No significant function in home
Needs prompting	Requires assistance in dressing, hygiene, keeping of personal effects	Requires much help with personal care; frequent incontinence

TABLE 3.10 Main features of the global deterioration scale[124]

Level	Clinical Characteristics
1 No cognitive decline	Normal; no subjective complaints or objective cognitive deficits
2 Very mild cognitive decline	Subjective memory complaints (misplacing items, forgetting well-known names) No impairment in social or occupational activities
3 Mild cognitive decline	Memory deficits evident to others, performance in demanding settings noticeably reduced Objective evidence of intensive interview (getting lost, prominent word-finding difficulties, poor short-term memory, lose valuable items)
4 Mild dementia	Clear deficits on clinical interview as demonstrated by decreased knowledge of current event, impaired serial subtractions, decreased ability to travel or handle finances Withdrawing from challenging social situations
5 Moderate dementia	No longer able to survive without some assistance
6 Moderately severe dementia	May forget spouse's name Largely unaware of recent events and experiences Generally unaware of surroundings Requires assistance with basic activities of daily living
7 Severe dementia	No verbal abilities Requires assistance in toileting and feeding Incontinent

Etiology of MCI: differential diagnosis

When memory complaints are of uncertain significance or when other disorders are present that may account for cognitive deficits, MCI (mild cognitive impairment) may reflect heterogeneous states. Broadly defined, the term may encompass the earliest changes of AD (Alzheimer's disease) or another non-AD dementia, non-demented persons with poor pre-morbid cognitive function, and healthy aging persons who are "worried-well" individuals.

"Worried-well"

Not all individuals with the diagnosis of MCI will progress to dementia and some may even improve over time. The "worried-well" represent a diagnostically challenging group of patients. While personal memory failures are common to everyone on a daily basis, the regularity of forgetfulness can be misleading to someone who is fearful of developing AD. These patients tend to have issues exacerbating their fears such as a family history of dementia, a history of depression, or psychosocial causes of stress. They typically self-report lapses in memory retrieval – such as temporarily forgetting a name or an item in the house they were pursuing – only to recall it some time later. Other typical complaints include word-finding difficulties in mid-conversation, brief episodes of geographic confusion in familiar places, or forgetting a highly routine activity such as locking a door or taking their medicine.

In contrast, incipient dementia is often accompanied by a loss of self-appreciation. Many individuals never acknowledge their memory impairment, but their impairments are usually quite apparent to knowledgeable family members or friends. Self-reported memory loss that is not verified by a collateral source can be an important clue to the nature of the memory complaints and raises the suspicion of "worried-well". On the other hand, low-grade cognitive impairment is not, on the whole, benign,[24] and these patients often require follow-up evaluations.

Depression

Memory complaints are a frequent symptom of depression, and depressed individuals may have a measurable decline in some aspects of memory.[125–128] The concept of pseudo-dementia arose to characterize depression as a potential mimic of dementia and highlight its reversibility with appropriate treatment.

The concept of pseudo-dementia, however, has been called into question.[129,130] Depression is frequently present in AD patients,[131,132] and patients diagnosed with pseudo-dementia frequently later develop diagnosable dementia.[133] In a prospective study, symptoms of depression were associated with an increased risk of developing AD.[134] With each additional depressive symptom, the risk of AD increased linearly by nearly 20%. Depression coexists with AD in up to 12% of demented patients. (add a reference to Forsell 1998 which is currently number 95 in the reference list) Cognitively normal older individuals who develop depression are at increased risk of developing subsequent mild cognitive impairment.[7,8] Depressive symptoms in individuals with AD have been related to pathology in the locus ceruleus and the substantia nigra,[135] suggesting that depression may be an early manifestation of AD or a dementia prodrome. We found little relation between three indices of depression and cognitive performance in AD.[100] These findings support the idea that depression is more often a predictor of dementia than it is an imitator.[130]

Depressive symptoms in early AD are associated with a more rapid rate of cognitive decline, suggesting that depression may interact with dementia to accelerate loss of functioning. Importantly, effectively treating depression can have an impact on the severity of cognitive-related disability as depression may interact with dementia to accelerate loss of functioning.[136] A low threshold for treatment of depressive symptoms in patients with cognitive impairment is important as some associated cognitive impairments may be reversed.[137]

Other etiologies

Other potential etiologies for memory complaints are important to highlight. Patients with long-standing inefficiencies in cognition may be identified after psychometric testing has revealed impaired function. Thus, patients at the low end of normal or who have had life-long cognitive difficulties may be included in study samples of MCI subjects, particularly if the criteria employed rely primarily on psychometric testing rather than history. Static, long-standing cognitive problems, rather than a change from the individual's previous level of functioning, do not imply subsequent deterioration unless a change from the individual's previous level of functioning is also present.

Structural brain lesions can lead to impairments in cognition, and therefore any change in cognition should be evaluated with appropriate imaging. Stroke, tumors, multiple sclerosis, intracerebral hemorrhage, subdural hemorrhage, chronic meningitis, and other infections (such as HIV) can all lead to cognitive changes. Systemic illness and medications can lead to changes in cognition, particularly delirium. Agents with anticholinergic properties are notorious for influencing cognition. Cardiovascular, respiratory, and metabolic derangements should be ruled out as possible causes of, or contributing factors in, memory impairment (Table 4.1).

Neurodegenerative dementias

In practice, MCI has come to represent a prodromal state of AD, given evidence from longitudinal studies indicating that individuals characterized as having amnestic MCI primarily progress to AD. Less common variants of MCI present with localized impairments in other cognitive domains while sparing memory. These variants may represent a prodrome of non-AD clinical syndromes such as frontotemporal dementia, dementia with Lewy bodies, or cortical basal degeneration.[81] Recognition of this heterogeneity has led to the proposal of other forms of MCI (Tables 4.2 and 4.3).

TABLE 4.1 Differential diagnosis of cognitive decline

- Neurodegenerative dementia
- Cerebrovascular disorders
    - Vascular dementia
    - Binswanger's disease
- Infectious disorders
    - Chronic meningitis
    - Encephalitis
        - Human Immunodeficiency virus
        - Lyme disease
    - Progressive multifocal leukoencephalopathy
    - Neurosyphilis
    - Whipple's disease
- Toxic/metabolic encephalopathies
    - Drugs/medications
    - Endocrine – thyroid, parathyroid
        - Nutritional – B12 and thiamine deficiecncies
        - Fluid and electrolyte abnormalities
        - Hypoglycemia
        - Other: carbon monoxide, heavy metals (lead, mercury, arsenic, thallium)
- Inflammatory
    - Vasculitis
        - Primary central nervous system vasculitis
        - Systemic vasculitides
            - Systemic lupus erythematosus
            - Polyarteritis nodosa
            - Wegener's granulomatosus
            - Churg-Strauss syndrome
        - Sarcoidosis
- Demyelinating
    - Multiple sclerosis
- Neoplastic
    - Direct effects of primary and metastatic disease
    - Paraneoplastic syndromes
- Hydrocephalus
- Affective disorders (depression)
- Neurogenetic disorders
    - Spinocerebellar ataxias
    - Dentatorubral-pallidoluysian atrophy
    - Hallervorden-Spatz disease
    - Gangliosidoses
    - Adult neuronal ceroid lipofuscinosis (Kuf's disease)
    - Mitochondrial encephalopathies
    - Porphyrias
    - Wilson's disease

TABLE 4.2 Neurodegenerative dementias

- Alzheimer's disease
- Dementia with Lewy bodies
- Vascular dementia
- Frontotemporal lobar degeneration
  - Frontotemporal dementia
  - Semantic aphasia
  - Progressive non-fluent apahsia
- Pick's disease
  - Progressive non-fluent aphasia
  - Semantic dementia
- Progressive supranuclear palsy
- Corticobasal degeneration
- Parkinson's disease with dementia
- Multiple system atrophy
- Huntington's disease
- Prion disorders
  - Creutzfeld-Jakob disease
  - Fatal familial insomnia
- Gerstmann-Straussler Scheinker disease

TABLE 4.3 Proposed forms of MCI[13]. Individuals with amnestic MCI appear to progress primarily to AD. Variants of MCI involving non-memory domains such as language, executive functioning and visuospatial skills may represent a prodrome to AD or other non-AD forms of dementia. Adapted with permission from Peterson (2001).[81]

Amnestic MCI →	Alzheimer's disease
Multiple domains slightly impaired →	Vascular dementia Normal Aging?
Single non-memory domain MCI →	Frontotemporal dementia Dementia with Lewy bodies Vascular dementia Parkinson's disease Alzheimer's disease

Overlap disorders

AD is often accompanied by other age-related disorders. Vascular lesions and Parkinson's disease most commonly coexist with AD, each occurring in about 25% of AD cases. "Pure" AD accounts for about 50–60% of clinically diagnosed cases of dementia. These concomitant disorders contribute to the expression of AD, as the histopathological burden of AD lesions for a given level of dementia severity is lower when AD is mixed with other disorders.[56,103,138] Given heterogeneity of clinical features and common pathological overlap, the true occurrence of the non-AD dementias is difficult to ascertain. Dementia with Lewy bodies, vascular dementia, and the frontotemporal dementias are considered the most common forms of non-AD dementias.

Dementia with Lewy bodies

Improvement in the pathological identification of Lewy bodies[139] has led to increasing appreciation that dementia with Lewy bodies (DLB) may be the second most frequent dementing illness after AD[140]. The term DLB characterizes a Parkinsonian syndrome in which neuropsychiatric disturbances are prominent. The clinical diagnosis of DLB requires the presence of dementia and at least one of three cardinal features: visual hallucinations, Parkinsonism, and fluctuating cognitive status. Consensus criteria[140] (Table 4.4) are recommended for making the diagnosis of DLB despite imperfect reliability and validity.[98] Greater frequency of extrapyramidal features and relatively better memory performance may characterize DLB as opposed to AD.

Pathologically, DLB is marked by the presence of intraneuronal Lewy bodies in regions such as the entorhinal cortex and the anterior cingulate cortex (Figure 4.1). Lewy bodies are also present in the substantia nigra, thus most cases also fulfill the neuropathological criteria for Parkinson's disease (PD). Considerable pathological overlap exists between DLB, AD, and PD. Most cases of DLB have concomitant lesions of AD with pure DLB pathology being rare. Most, if not all, cases of PD have cortical Lewy bodies, and around

TABLE 4.4 Dementia with Lewy bodies. 1996 Consensus Criteria for the Clinical Diagnosis[140]

1. Dementia (required central feature)
   a. Prominent memory impairment may not necessarily occur in the early stages but is usually evident with progression
   b. Deficits in attention, frontal-subcortical skills, and visuospatial abilities may be especially prominent
2. Two of the following core features must be present for a diagnosis of probable DLB, one for possible DLB:
   a. Fluctuating cognition with pronounced variations in attention and alertness
   b. Recurrent visual hallucinations that are typically well formed and detailed
   c. Spontaneous motor features of parkinsonism
3. Features supportive of the diagnosis
   a. Repeated falls
   b. Syncope
   c. Transient loss of consciousness
   d. Neuroleptic sensitivity
   e. Systematized delusions
   f. Hallucinations in other modalities
4. A diagnosis of DLB is less likely in the presence of
   a. Stroke disease, evident as focal neurologic signs or on brain imaging
   b. Evidence on physical examination and investigation of any physical illness or other brain disorder sufficient to account for the picture

25% of PD patients eventually become demented.[141] The clinical relevance of cortical Lewy bodies and the relationship of DLB to AD needs better understanding.

Vascular dementia

Vascular dementia appears to be overdiagnosed clinically, at least in the U.S.A.[142] Not only have most studies of vascular dementia in the U.S.A. not been supported by neuropathological confirmation, but those that have been studied often reveal the unexpected presence of AD with or without concomitant strokes.[143,144] Pure cases of vascular dementia are rare. A survey of 1,929 autopsied cases of dementia found only six with a pure vascular dementia.[145]

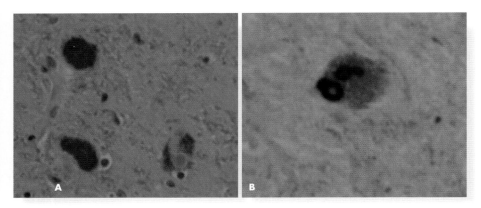

FIGURE 4.1 (A) Classic Lewy body in a pigmented dopaminergic cell of the substantia nigra. A densely eosinophilic center with a pale halo is characteristic of the classic Lewy body. **(B)** The Lewy body stains intensely with immunostaining for alpha synuclein.

The most clinically relevant issue with vascular dementia is likely to be the extent to which it interacts additively or synergistically with AD to produce dementia. The few clinicopathological studies of mixed dementia indicate that cerebrovascular lesions have an important role in contributing to AD onset and severity.[56,103] The modified Hachinski Ischemic Score[146] (Table 4.5) may be useful in identifying the majority of dementia patients with at least some cerebrovascular pathology.[98] (Figure 4.2)

Frontotemporal lobar dementias

Frontotemporal lobar dementias are characterized by disturbed personality, behavior, and language[147] reflecting the predominant pathological involvement of the prefrontal cortex and anterior temporal lobes. Frontotemporal lobar degeneration refers to circumscribed degeneration of the frontotemporal lobes with the associated clinical syndromes being determined by the anatomic distribution of the pathology (Figure 4.2).

The frontotemporal lobar-degeneration syndromes have been classified into three disorders[147] based on clinical presentation: frontotemporal dementia (FTD), semantic dementia, and progressive

TABLE 4.5 Modified Hachinski ischemic score

Feature	Present	Absent
Abrupt onset	2	0
Fluctuating course	2	0
History of strokes	2	0
Focal neurological signs	2	0
Focal neurological symptoms	2	0
Stepwise deterioration	1	0
Nocturnal confusion	1	0
Relative preservation of personality	1	0
Depression	1	0
Somatic complaints	1	0
Emotional incontinence	1	0
Hypertension	1	0
Evidence of atherosclerosis	1	0

A score of 7 or more is consistent with cerebrovascular pathology.

non-fluent aphasia (Table 4.6). The syndromes are predominantly pre-senile, occurring frequently before 65 years of age, and are often familial.[148] In a prevalence study of early-onset dementia, FTD was as common as AD with a mean age at onset of 58 years.[149]

The clinical symptoms of FTD include early behavioral dysfunction with disinhibition, impulsivity, impaired judgment, and disturbed social comportment. Severe amnesia and visuospatial impairment are typically not present. Progressive non-fluent aphasia is characterized by early loss of fluent speech and prominent anomie. Semantic aphasia is marked by early impairment in semantics (word meaning) resulting in empty, fluent speech and a loss of speech comprehension. The three syndromes tend to overlap and, as each disease progresses, the clinical symptoms will converge as progression results in eventual muteness and behavioral disturbance. Similar features can occur with AD, but are typically less pronounced and occur later in the course.

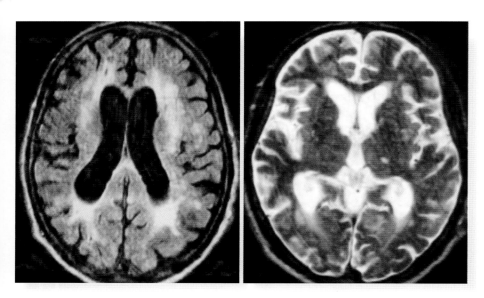

A Image and path

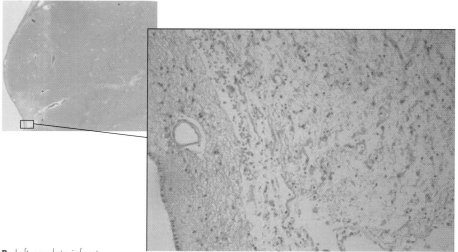

B Left caudate infarct

FIGURE 4.2 A 75 year old African American male had a progressive, gradual decline in cognition that began at the age of 69 with symptoms including difficulty driving, misplacing items and reduced judgment and problem solving. His symptoms progressed gradually in the ensuing 8 years. His medical history was notable during this time for the occurrence of several transient ischemic attacks. An MRI two weeks before death **(A)** for fever and unresponsiveness revealed significant white matter

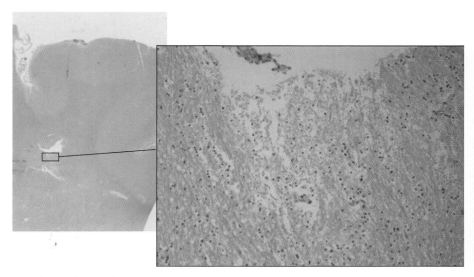

C Right frontal microinfarct

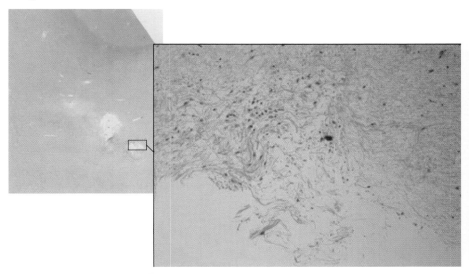

D Right parietal white matter infarct

changes and an infarct in the left thalamus. At the time of death from sepsis and cachexia, he was judged to have severe Alzheimer's dementia with cerebrovascular disease (CDR 3).
Neuropathological examination revealed the absence of amyloid plaques and tangles in the cortex and multiple infarcts in the basal ganglia and white matter **(B,C, and D)**.

TABLE 4.6 Frontotemporal lobar degenerations: clinical criteria[147]

	Frontotemporal dementia	Progressive non-fluent aphasia	Semantic dementia
Core Features	1. Decline in social personal conduct 2. Blunted emotions 3. Lack of insight	1. Non-fluent speech with prominent anomia, agrammatism, and paraphasias	1. Fluent speech lacking meaning 2. Prominent comprehension difficulties 3. Preserved drawing reproduction, single-word repetition, ability to read aloud and write to dictations
Supportive Features	• Decline in personal hygiene • Dietary changes • Preseverative • Stereotyped behavior • Late mutism	• Stuttering • Alexia • Agraphia • Late behavioral changes	• Pressured speech • Loss of sympathy or empathy

Pick's disease, the prototypical FTD, is characterized pathologically by the presence of Pick bodies, tau-positive neuronal inclusions, and severe neuronal loss, spongiform change and gliosis in the frontal and temporal cortex. More common presentations of FTD resemble Pick's disease clinically, except that neuronal inclusions are absent.

Abnormal forms of tau characterize other neurodegenerative disorders, including progressive supranuclear palsy and corticobasal degeneration.[150] These disorders often clinically resemble FTD, but occasionally mimic AD. Considerable pathological and clinical overlap may relate to different biochemical effects of mutations in *tau* or in other genes not yet identified.[151] The term Pick complex has been suggested as a unifying concept for these overlapping clinical disorders (Table 4.6, Figures 4.3, 4.4, 4.5).[152]

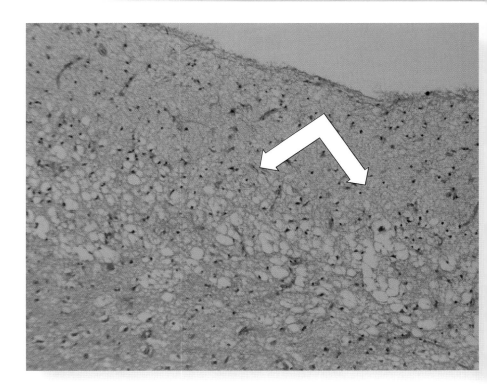

FIGURE 4.3 Frontal cortex from an individual with a clinical diagnosis of frontotemporal dementia. Neuropathological findings included severe neuronal loss with a spongiform changes in deep layers of the frontal cortex. Neuronal inclusions were absent. Photomicrograph courtesy of Daniel McKeel, MD, Washington University, St. Louis, U.S.A.

Identifying the subset of MCI that is AD

Our experience has indicated that clinical methods can accurately identify the subset within MCI for which AD is the responsible disorder.[72] These clinical methods rest on a reliable informant's report of consistent change from past levels of cognitive ability that interfere, albeit mildly, with usual activities. The diagnosis is made independent of neuropsychological assessments, such as the mini-mental state examination, because individual performance differences on cognitive measure may obscure the distinction between non-demented aging and very mild AD.

Information is gathered primarily through interviewing the informant in order to probe for evidence of the gradual onset and progression of cognitive decline compromising the patient's ability to carry out their accustomed activities. Older adults are not homogenous, and their everyday accustomed activities are quite variable. The collateral source's observations inform whether "instrumental" activities (e.g. driving, shopping, home repairs, cooking, handling finances) that are customary for the patient are being performed less well. This information is sensitive to changes in the patient's current cognitive performance in relation to previous abilities and is more sensitive to early dementia than cognitive test performance.[32–36] The wide range in performance of normal individuals, combined with variability introduced by factors such as education and race, limits the utility of cognitive tests, particularly with a single time of testing. Moreover, in individuals with superior baseline intellectual function who may still score in the normative range on cognitive measures, the collateral source-based method is sensitive to mild dementia.

While the exclusion of structural brain disease, hypothyroidism and other medical illnesses is important, the diagnosis of AD can be confidently made when the history suggests a slowly progressive deterioration of cognitive skills and the neurological examination is otherwise normal. Longitudinal studies suggest that these methods allow the accurate diagnosis of AD in patients with minimal impairments, many of whom have less cognitive impairment than that required for the diagnosis of MCI.[72] Previous studies have shown that very slight deficits in performance of daily activities (occasional reminding or assistance) are commonly observed in incipient AD for up to 2 years before diagnosis.[153]

The accurate and reliable identification of individuals with the earliest forms of AD is possible for several reasons. First, clinicians should expect cognitive function in truly non-demented individuals to be relatively stable with aging.[50,51,53–55] Memory failure should not be accepted as a normal part of aging; instead, in the absence of disease, relatively stable cognitive performance can be expected. Thus, even mild impairment is considered abnormal. Second, the

A   **B**

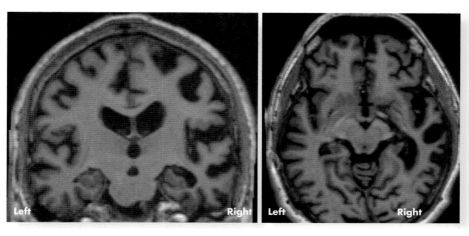

FIGURE 4.4 Coronal **(A)** and transverse **(B)** MRI of a 73 year old right handed man with 3 year history of progressive memory impairment and behavioral changes. The MRI revealed significant global atrophy most prominent in the right frontal and temporal lobes. His symptoms began with cognitive decline (difficulty balancing checkbook, repeating questions) and were accompanied by significant behavioral changes. Early feature include suspiciousness and paranoid delusions, socially inappropriate behavior, distractibility, and severe apathy. He was diagnosed with frontotemporal dementia. (Courtesy of Randy Buckner)

determination of "impairment" is operationalized as interference with performance of activities of daily living. This criterion requires the activities to simply be performed less well than before and not be fully relinquished. Third, our assessment importantly relies primarily on an informant's observations to identify early cognitive change and functional impairment.

Obtaining a clear history from a knowledgeable informant is, at the current time, the most sensitive means of detecting the earliest changes of a dementing illness. Psychometric testing and dementia-screening tools, such as the MMSE and the clock-drawing test, are insensitive to early changes of AD and other dementias. These tests should not be relied upon in making, or excluding, an early diagnosis of AD or a dementing illness. Indeed, a standard history and physical examination – utilizing the insight of a knowledgeable family member or friend – cannot be replaced.

Treatment of MCI and dementia

As many individuals with MCI (mild cognitive impairment) are likely to have early AD (Alzheimer's disease), utilization of therapies for AD may be applicable. There are few data at present, however, to support treatment in MCI. The U.S. Food and Drug Administration has approved pharmacological treatment of mild to moderate AD with cholinesterase inhibitors, and moderate to severe AD with the NMDA (*N*-methyl-D-aspartate)-antagonist memantine.

Clinical trials are in progress to evaluate the effectiveness of several agents in preventing or slowing the rate of "conversion" from MCI to dementia. The Alzheimer's Disease Cooperative Study is conducting a randomized controlled trial to assess vitamin E and donepezil in delaying the clinical progression from MCI to AD. The National Institute of Mental Health is comparing ibuprofen with placebo in patients with age-associated memory impairment as defined by poor performance on verbal memory, visual memory, and verbal fluency. The Investigation into the Delay to Diagnosis of Alzheimer's disease with Exelon study is a multicenter randomized, placebo-controlled trial assessing the effect of rivastigmine on patients with MCI. These and other medications may eventually be approved for the symptomatic treatment, prevention, or delay in progression of MCI. Currently, however, no medications are approved for treatment of MCI, and there is little consensus on when to begin therapy (Table 5.1).

MCI

The case for early treatment

Although little consensus exists on when to begin treatment in patients with cognitive changes, there is a growing trend towards treating cognitive decline increasingly early. This trend is stimulated by the improved ability of clinicians to detect early-stage AD and

TABLE 5.1 MCI trials: preventing development or worsening of AD

- Cholinergic Drugs
  - Rivastigmine
  - Galantamine
  - Donepezil
  - Donepezil +/- gingko biloba
- Glutamatergic drugs
  - CX516 (Ampalex) – AMPA agonist
- Anti-inflammatory
  - Ibuprofen
  - Celecoxib
- Estrogen
- Antioxidants
  - Gingko biloba
  - Vitamin E and selenium
- Cholesterol-reducing agents

the recognition that a majority of individuals with MCI probably have early AD.

Data generated from open-label trials have suggested a potential benefit from the use of cholinesterase inhibitors early in the course of AD. In these trials,[154,155] individuals initially randomized to placebo and then subsequently treated with open-label drugs benefited from cholinesterase inhibitors, but never to the same degree experienced by people randomized to the drugs from the start. These observations offer tentative support for the theory that treatment early in the disease course may lead to greater benefit and potentially delay cognitive decline (Figures 5.1 and 5.2).

There are several caveats regarding pharmacological treatment of patients with MCI. First, long-term benefits from early treatment with cholinesterase inhibitors have not been clearly demonstrated, although treatment does provide limited symptomatic benefit.[11] In addition, the potential for unidentified harm from taking unnecessary or unproven medications exists, although no serious

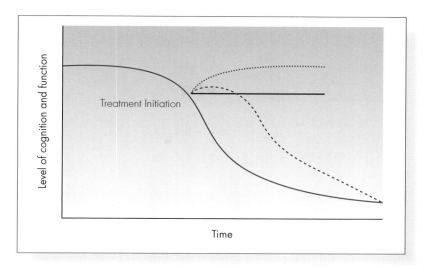

FIGURE 5.1 Hypothetical treatment responses. Treatment of AD would ideally return the individual to prior levels of cognition and function, restoring all lost abilities (·········· line). Alternatively, treatment may halt future disease progression, allowing the individual to remain at their current level of functioning (black line). In reality, current treatment temporarily halts decline or slightly improves function for up to 1 year before the symptomatic progression resumes its downward trend. There is no apparent effect on underlying disease progression.

toxicities have been identified from cholinesterase inhibitors that would warrant avoidance of treatment.

Our current practice is to begin symptomatic therapy as soon as cognitive decline interfering with function is identified. Early treatment offers symptomatic benefit at low risk of adverse side effects. Moreover, the recognition and treatment of MCI as early-stage dementia allows patients to be involved in planning their future care at a stage when they still retain decisional capacity.

Non-pharmacological treatment

There are non-pharmacological treatments of MCI that may be of some benefit. For instance, there is evidence suggesting that physical and leisure activities, as well as mentally stimulating activities, decrease the rate of cognitive decline in non-demented adults and the

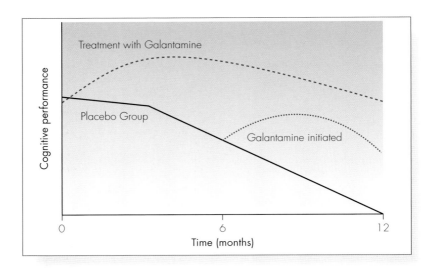

FIGURE 5.2 In a trial assessing Galantamine in AD,[154] patients receiving active drug (red line) sustained mild improvement in cognitive testing over 1 year, while those receiving placebo (*black line*) worsened at a predictable rate. A subset of those who received placebo for the first 6 months were given open-label active medication for the subsequent 6 months (·············· *line*). Their cognitive scores never improved to the level of those receiving active drug during the entire trial. These open-label data suggest earlier treatment with cholinesterase inhibitors may be beneficial. Further research is needed, however, to verify these speculative results. Reproduced from Neurology 2000, 54: 2261–2268, with permission from Lippincott Williams and Wilkins.[154]

risk of AD.[156,157] For instance, in a prospective study of 469 non-demented subjects, participation in leisure activities (including reading, playing board games, playing musical instruments, and dancing) were associated with a reduced risk of dementia. Additionally, in a study of 437 subjects over the age of 75, baseline level of leisure activities was associated with a lower risk of developing mild cognitive impairment.[9] Thus, there is some evidence to support the recommendation of increased physical and mental activity for MCI individuals.

Other non-pharmacological interventions include recognizing the effects that stress, decreased sleep, and medications (i.e. sedatives and anticholinergic drugs) can have on memory function, and removing these influences. Additionally, vascular risk factors should be aggressively treated as they have been shown to interact with the clinical expression of AD.[103]

In counseling the patient with MCI, the statistical risk for progression to further stages of impairment should be noted; however, there clearly exist subsets of MCI patients who never progress, and many individuals with MCI improve to normal over follow up.[24] The patient should be seen routinely for follow-up assessments in order to monitor for progression.[112]

Dementia therapy

As many patients with MCI in actuality have early AD, we will review current dementia therapy and explore possible future pharmacological strategies. Advances in our understanding of the neurobiological mechanisms underlying AD, primarily the cholinergic and amyloid hypotheses, have stimulated efforts at developing disease-modifying agents that may potentially halt progression or even prevent development of disease.

Approved therapies

Cholinergic hypothesis

The observation of a consistent and profound acetylcholine deficit in the brains of individuals with AD led to the generation of the cholinergic hypothesis. The hypothesis states that selective degeneration of basal forebrain cholinergic neurons in AD results in a cerebral cholinergic deficit; this underlies the characteristic memory impairment.[158] Several lines of evidence implicate impaired cholinergic transmission in contributing to the symptoms of AD. This includes observations of memory and attention deficits resulting from lesions of basal forebrain neurons and pharmacological blockade of muscarinic acetylcholine receptors. Additionally, neocortical and hippocampal acetyl cholinesterase activity and cholinergic cell number is consistently reduced in the brains of AD patients (Figure 5.3).[73]

Emerging evidence from post-mortem studies of individuals in mild stages of AD, however, challenges the cholinergic hypothesis. Depletion of the cholinergic marker, choline acetyltransferase, is

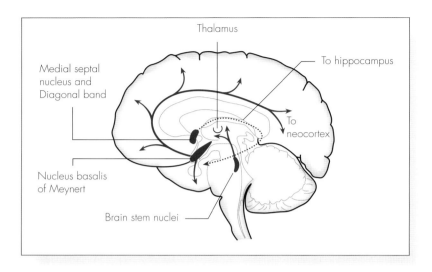

FIGURE 5.3 The basal nucleus of Meynert in the basal forebrain gives rise to widespread cholinergic neurons innervating most of the cerebral cortex. AD brains have consistently demonstrated reduced numbers of cholinergic cells in the basal forebrain and lowered acetylcholine enzymatic activity throughout the cortex. The cholinergic hypothesis posits that selective degeneration of the basal forebrain cholinergic neurons results in a cholinergic deficit that contributes to AD symptoms. The cholinergic hypothesis has provided a rationale for the development of effective treatment in ameliorating the symptoms of AD.

found only in end-stage but not in mild to moderate AD[159,160] or in MCI.[73] These findings cast doubt on the relevance of the cholinergic hypothesis for the initial stages of AD, and suggest that mechanisms other than simple cholinergic "replacement" may be involved in the modest efficacy demonstrated by the cholinesterase inhibitors.

Despite recent challenges, the cholinergic hypothesis has provided a rationale for developing symptomatic treatment for AD.[161] The drug discovery and clinical trial efforts based on this hypothesis have pioneered the development of drugs that successfully ameliorate the symptoms of AD. Centrally acting cholinesterase inhibitors represent the first agents to be approved by the U.S. Food and Drug Administration for the symptomatic treatment of AD (Figure 5.4).

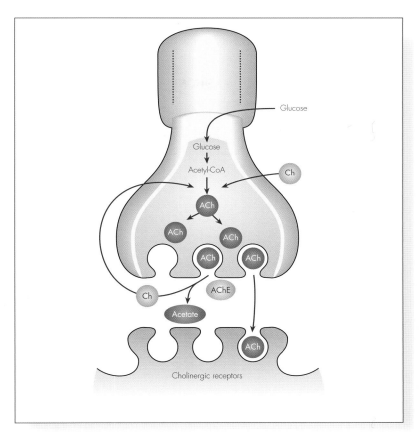

FIGURE 5.4 After release into the synapse, acetylcholine (ACh) is degraded by the enzyme acetylcholinesterase (AChE) into choline (Ch) and acetate. Inhibition of the enzyme acetylcholinesterase reduces the metabolism of acetylcholine, effectively increasing the concentration of acetylcholine in the synapse. Acetylcholinesterase inhibitors are currently the cornerstone of symptomatic treatment of AD.

Cholinesterase inhibitors

Cholinesterase inhibitors are currently the cornerstone of symptomatic treatment of AD. There are currently four approved drugs in the U.S.A.: tacrine, donepezil, rivastigmine, and galantamine. Tacrine is considered a first-generation cholinesterase inhibitor and is no longer prescribed due to adverse effects. Newer-generation drugs have advantages that permit easier administration and a reduced adverse-effect profile (Table 5.2).

Multiple trials[154,162–172] have demonstrated a modest but significant benefit from cholinesterase inhibitors with a treatment effect that appears to last at least 1 year. AD patients treated with cholinesterase inhibitors do better overall on tests of cognition than those treated with placebo. Additionally, deteriorations in ability to perform

TABLE 5.2 Dosing and tolerability of cholinesterase inhibitors

	Trial completion (5–6-month trials)*		Discontinuation related to adverse events*		Dosing		
	Active	Placebo	Active	Placebo	Frequency	Initial Dose	Dose Escalation†
Donepezil 253,254	68–85%	80%	6–18%	7–10%	Once daily	5 mg QD	Additional 5 mg after 4–6 weeks, as tolerated, up to 10 mg
Rivastigmine 166,169	63–86%	82–87%	7–29%	7%	Twice daily	1.5 mg BID	Additional 3 mg (1.5 mg BID) every two weeks, as tolerated, up to 6–12 mg total daily dose
Galantamine 154,255	68–78%	81–84%	6–23%	7–8%	Twice daily	4 mg BID	Additional 8 mg (4 mg BID) every 4 weeks, as tolerated, up to 16–24 mg total daily dose

* Reported ranges reflect differences across trials, various doses and dose escalation schedules.
† Dose escalation recommendations have been taken from the medication package inserts. Others may find different dose escalation schedules (i.e. slower titration schedule) to be better tolerated.

activities of daily living are less in those treated with active medication. Economic models indicate that cholinesterase inhibitors may increase the period before patients require long-term care. The associated reductions in health-care expenditures offset the costs of drugs and result in overall savings.[173]

An evidenced-based review of the management of dementia[174] concluded that a measurable benefit in cognition, behavior, and functioning occurs with the use of this class of drugs, although the size of the effect is small. The goal of cholinesterase-inhibitor therapy is primarily one of maintenance of memory, cognition, mood and behavior. Symptomatic progression of the disease may be delayed for at least 12 months, although there is no apparent effect on underlying disease progression. In addition, the cholinesterase inhibitors are well tolerated, and their use has been shown to be cost-effective. These data suggest that cholinesterase inhibitors generally are well tolerated and may enable patients to remain for at least 1 year at or near their level of function at the time of drug initiation.

Donepezil

Donepezil (Aricept™) became the second drug, after tacrine, to be approved for treatment of the cognitive symptoms of AD. Donepezil is a piperidine-based reversible cholinesterase inhibitor that is highly selective for CNS (central nervous system) acetylcholinesterase. The efficacy of donepezil therapy has been shown across multiple double-blind, placebo-controlled, multicenter trials demonstrating benefits in function, behavior, and cognitive performance for mild to moderate AD.

There is data to suggest some limited symptomatic benefit of Donepezil in patients with MCI. In a study of 769 subjects with mild cognitive impairment, Donepezil was associated with a lower rate of progression to AD during the first 12 months of treatment, although there was no difference in the study's primary outcome measure of rate of progression to AD over three years. Overall cognitive function of the MCI subjects in the Donepezil group did not decline on most measures during the first 6–18 months, but declined thereafter at the same rate as the placebo group. This study provides modest evidence that treatment with Donepezil may delay the clinical diagnosis of AD and have a symptomatic effect on cognitive symptoms of MCI.[11]

Donepezil's long half-life supports once-daily administration, and there is no requirement for dose modifications in the elderly or in patients with renal or hepatic impairment. Donepezil is generally well tolerated, particularly with dose titration. Initiation of therapy is recommended at 5 mg/day, given at bedtime, with dose escalation to 10 mg/day after at least 2 weeks. The higher dose is associated with a higher frequency of side effects, namely diarrhea and vomiting, although these adverse effects are generally mild and brief, and are often avoidable with dose titration.

Rivastigmine

Rivastigmine (Exelon™) is a long-acting reversible, non-competitive carbamate acetylcholinesterase inhibitor, designed to inhibit both brain forms of cholinesterase – aceytlcholinesterase and butyrylcholinesterase. Acetylcholinesterase makes up the majority of cholinesterase and functions primarily in the synapses throughout the nervous system. Butyrylcholinesterase is of glial origin and has more general actions in the brain that are not well-understood. As AD progresses and cortical neurons are lost, levels of acetylcholinesterase decline, while butyrylcholinesterase levels increase and take over function metabolizing acetylcholine at the synapse.

Efficacy in treating the cognitive symptoms of AD has been demonstrated in a prospective, randomized, multicenter, double-blind, placebo-controlled trial. The starting dose of rivastigmine is 1.5 mg twice a day. If this dose is well tolerated for at least 2 weeks, the dose may be increased to 3 mg twice daily, with subsequent increases to 4.5 mg and 6 mg after a minimum of 2 weeks at the previous dose. As with the other cholinesterase inhibitors, the most common adverse events are largely cholinergic effects such as nausea, vomiting, and anorexia. These side effects are largely avoidable with dose titration.

Galantamine

Galantamine (Razadyne™) is a tertiary alkaloid derived originally from the *Amyryllidaceae* family of plants, which include daffodils and the common snowdrop. Galantamine is a reversible inhibitor of acetylcholinesterase that acts by binding to the active site of acetylcholinesterase, thereby inhibiting the enzyme. It has additional agonist properties at nicotinic receptors; these properties have been speculated to provide an additional therapeutic mechanism by acting synergistically with acetylcholine to facilitate nicotinic acetylcholine receptors.

The effectiveness of galantamine has been demonstrated in at least four large placebo-controlled trials to improve the cognitive and behavioral symptoms of AD. The recommended starting dose of galantamine is 4 mg twice a day. After a minimum of 4 weeks of treatment, if tolerated, the dose should be increased to 8 mg twice a day (16 mg/day), with a further increase to 12 mg twice a day (24 mg/day) after a minimum of 4 weeks at the previous dose.

Memantine

Memantine was approved for the treatment of moderate to severe AD in the U.S.A. in late 2003. It has received marketing authorization in Europe for the treatment of moderately severe to severe AD and is the standard pharmacotherapy for AD in Germany.

The rationale for memantine's neuroprotective effect is its ability to block the N-methyl-D-aspartate (NMDA) glutamate receptor, which may play a role in excitotoxicity. Processes such as ischemia, trauma, and hypoglycemia may induce cell death by increasing the sensitivity of the glutamate receptors. Excitotoxic neuronal damage as a result of chronic glutamatergic overstimulation has been postulated as a common mechanism underlying neurodegenerative diseases.[175] The post-synaptic glutamate receptor NMDA has been implicated in the pathogenesis of AD[176] and may be a promising target for neuroprotective agents. Aβ's toxic effects may, in part, be mediated by glutamate production, resulting in enhancement of the NMDA receptor and subsequent excitotoxic effects (Figure 5.5).[177]

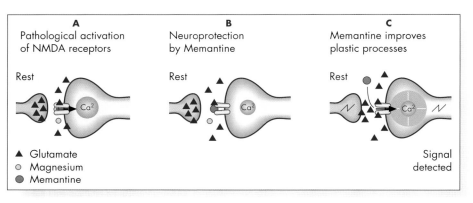

FIGURE 5.5 The NMDA receptor may have an excitotoxic role in processes such as ischemia, trauma, hypoglycemia, and neurodegenerative disorders **(A)**. The higher calcium permeability of this receptor in these conditions may underlie its neurotoxic potential. Memantine is an NMDA antagonist that may act to reduce excess Ca^{2+} permeability of the NMDA receptor in resting condition **(B)**. Memantine's reversible binding to the receptor may allow relevant physiologic signals to be detected **(C)**.Used with permission Danysz et al.

The first multi-center trial in the U.S.A. of memantine in moderate to advanced AD suggested that memantine is safe, well-tolerated, and may be modestly efficacious in slowing the rate of deterioration of moderate to severe AD.[178] In this double-blind, placebo-controlled clinical trial of 28 weeks duration, 252 subjects (mean age 75 years, mean MMSE score 7.9) were randomized to receive either Memantine 20 mg/day or placebo. Both treatment groups experienced decline in the primary outcome measures over the course of the study; however, the memantine-treated individuals deteriorated more slowly, as judged by the physician, and in their functional performance. Additionally, the required care-giver time for the memantine-treated group was significantly less than for the placebo group. Memantine appeared to be safe and well-tolerated. The frequency of reported adverse events did not differ significantly between memantine and placebo.[178]

Memantine in combination with the cholinesterase inhibitor donepezil has been shown to result in improved cognitive, functional, and behavioral outcomes compared with the use of donepezil alone in a 24-week trial. Combining donepezil and memantine, which work on different neurotransmitter systems, may bestow each agent's independent clinical benefits, thereby leading to an additive or synergistic effect.[179]

The role of memantine in treating early-stage AD is unclear. The results of efficacy studies testing memantine in mild-to-moderate AD patients have not yet been reported. Until this information is available, the full role of memantine in the pharmacotherapy of AD remains to be determined.

Agents under investigation for AD treatment and prevention

Multiple agents are under investigation for potential use in preventing AD and for treatment once AD has been diagnosed. Amyloid (Aβ) accumulation appears to have synaptotoxic and neurodegenerative effects. Numerous approaches have been postulated to provide protection from these effects, including antioxidant, neuroprotective, or neurotrophic properties.

Vitamin E and selegeline

Alpha-tocopherol (Vitamin E; 1,000 IU twice daily) is an antioxidant that has been shown in a randomized controlled trial to delay progression to clinical markers of dementia in moderately demented AD patients.[180] In the same study, selegeline (5 mg BID), a monoamine oxidase inhibitor, also delayed progression, although the combination of selegeline and vitamin E yielded no additive or synergistic effect. Neither drug improved cognitive function. The 2001 AAN practice parameter on the treatment of dementia recommends Vitamin E potentially to slow AD progression.[174] Selegeline has a less favorable risk–benefit ratio than vitamin E and was not recommended for routine use in AD therapy.

Vitamin E in combination with vitamin C is associated with reduced prevalence and incidence of AD. In a population-based, observational study of 4,740 subjects participating in the Cache County Study, combined use of vitamin E and C supplements was associated with a 78% reduction in the risk of having AD at study onset (prevalence) and a 64% reduced risk of developing AD during the 3 years of follow up.[181] This study suggests a possible role for vitamin E in combination with vitamin C for the primary prevention of AD. Randomized controlled trials, however, are necessary to prove the efficacy of these agents.

Despite this, there appears to be little evidence to recommend Vitamin E for the treatement of MCI. In a randomized controlled of trial of vitamin E and donepezil in patients with MCI, there were no benefits of 2000 IU of vitamin E in patients with MCI. Those treated with vitamin E showed no decreased risk of progression to AD or benefits in cognitive testing over this time period.[11]

Estrogen

There is a strong biological basis for using estrogen therapy as a potential strategy for preventing dementia and AD. Estrogen has been shown to have neurotrophic effects, reduce $A\beta$ accumulation, enhance neurotransmitter release and action, and provide protection against oxidative damage.[182] Additionally, prospective and case-control studies have reported a lower risk of developing AD in women taking estrogen.[183–186]

These findings, however, have recently been called into question. In the Women's Health Initiative 4,532 women were randomized to either placebo or 0.625 mg of conjugated estrogen and 2.5 mg of medroxyprogesterone acetate. After an average of 4 years of follow-up, the hazard ratio of developing dementia was two times higher in those treated with estrogen and progesterone compared with placebo.[187] Additionally, women in the treatment group had a slightly increased likelihood of declining on cognitive testing[188] and were 31% more likely to have stroke.[189] In 2002, the estrogen and progestin treatment arm of the Women's Health Initiative was stopped prematurely because treatment was associated with a significantly increased risk of coronary heart disease, stroke, pulmonary embolus, and breast cancer.[190] In 2004, the estrogen-only arm of the Women's Health Initiative was also stopped prematurely. After 7 years of follow-up estrogen alone was associated with an increased risk of stroke and an absence of benefit for cardiovascular risks. Additionally, estrogen alone does not protect against the development of dementia: 47 participants developed dementia, 28 an estrogen-alone and 19 a placebo. Thus, estrogen alone or estrogen combined with progestin therapy cannot be recommended for prevention of any outcome.

Anti-inflammatory agents

The pathophysiology of AD may, in part, be related to inflammation.[191] This has been suggested by biochemical and neuropathological data indicating that Aβ accumulation induces an inflammatory response in the cortex that may damage neurons and exacerbate the neuropathological processes underlying the disease. Elevated inflammatory cytokines have been measured in AD patients[192] and in patients with cognitive decline.[193] Thus, anti-inflammatory medications may provide neuroprotective benefits.

Observational studies have suggested reduced risk of developing AD in those taking anti-inflammatory drugs,[194,195] although no definitive preventive study results have been published. A large population-based study of 6,989 subjects found those on long-term anti-inflammatory medications had an up to 80% reduction in the risk of developing AD. The reduction in risk of developing AD was less for those taking anti-inflammatory medications for shorter periods of time, suggesting a dose-dependent effect.[195] A second rationale for the potential usefulness of anti-inflammatory medications in preventing AD come from a study demonstrating that some anti-inflammatory medications decrease the production of Aβ in cultured cells. Thus, anti-inflammatory medications may potentially have a direct effect on amyloid pathology in the brain.[194]

There is little evidence to support the use of anti-inflammatory drugs in the treatment of AD at this time. The largest study of prednisone on the treatment of AD was negative.[196] A trial of ibuprofen in age-associated memory impairment is ongoing. The intriguing results of observational studies must be replicated in prospective primary prevention trials before anti-inflammatory medications can be recommended in the treatment or prevention of AD.

Cholesterol-reducing agents

There is increasing interest in the potential use of statins for treatment or prevention of AD. Two observational studies in individuals using lipid-lowering agents have reported a 40–79% reduction in the risk of dementia[197] and AD.[198] Biochemical data suggest a relationship between cholesterol, the processing of the amyloid precursor protein, and the risk of AD.[199] Though statins have a proposed role in reducing amyloid production, prospective trials are needed before they can be recommended as symptomatic or preventive AD therapy.

Chelation therapy

$A\beta$ aggregation appears to be, in part, dependent on Cu^{2+} and Zn^{2+} metal ions. Reduced $A\beta$ deposition has been observed in *APP* (amyloid precursor protein) transgenic mice treated with the antibiotic clioquinol, a known Cu^{2+} and Zn^{2+} chelator.[200] Clioquinol was withdrawn from the market in 1970 for its association with subacute myelo-optic neuropathy, possibly related to Vitamin B12 deficiency. It was recently re-evaluated[201] in a pilot study in which 36 subjects with AD were randomized to either placebo or clioquinol. In this small sample, clioquinol was generally well tolerated, and the treatment group had minimal cognitive deterioration, reduced plasma $A\beta$, and elevated plasma Zn^{2+} levels compared with the placebo group. Further trials are warranted and necessary to explore the potential use of clioquinol in AD. The data are not yet sufficient to support the use of clioquinol in AD at the present time.

Future therapeutic and diagnostic strategies

Amyloid hypothesis

The amyloid hypothesis speculates that accumulation of beta-amyloid protein (Aβ) is the critical trigger leading to pathological changes in the brains of AD (Alzheimer's disease) patients.[202] The hypothesis states that insoluble Aβ accumulation initiates a cascade of events, resulting in synapse loss, activation of inflammatory processes, induction of neurofibrillary changes, and ultimately neuronal death (Figure 6.1).

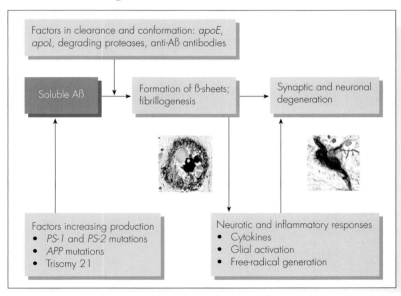

FIGURE 6.1 The amyloid hypotheis states that accumulation of beta-amyloid (Aβ) is central in the pathogenesis of AD. Factors increasing Aβ production, changing its conformation, or reducing its clearance lead to Aβ aggregation in insoluble clumps of β-sheets. These aggregations appear to have direct and indirect neurotoxic and inflammatory effects that lead to synaptic and neuronal degeneration. Modified from David M. Holtzman MD, Washington University, St. Louis, U.S.A.

The source of Aβ appears to be alternative processing of the amyloid precursor protein (APP). APP is a ubiquitously expressed protein. Though its function is still unknown, it appears to be a membrane-spanning protein. The processing of APP is complex. Processing occurs through several routes, one of which can lead to the abnormal production and accumulation of Aβ. Normally, APP is cleaved by alpha-secretase such that the Aβ peptide is not produced. Alternative sequential proteolytic cleavage of APP by beta- and gamma-secretase, however, generates intact Aβ in two lengths, either $A\beta_{1-40}$ or $A\beta_{1-42}$. If peptide production exceeds clearance capacity, these peptides aggregate and form insoluble deposits (diffuse plaques) in the neocortex. Factors increasing alternative APP processing over its basal levels or affecting its cerebral clearance result in Aβ deposition that may be the critical initiating step in the pathogenesis of AD (Figure 6.2).

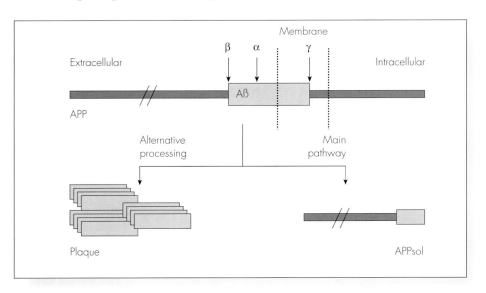

FIGURE 6.2 Processing of amyloid precursor protein. Amyloid precursor protein (APP) is a ubiquitous membrane-spanning protein of unknown function. Abnormal processing of APP appears to be the source of beta-amyloid (Aβ). Normal processing of APP occurs with alpha-secretase cleaving near the center of Aβ, such that Aβ is not produced. The alternative pathway involves beta- and gamma secretases cleaving Aβ from APP. This pathway appears to generate intact Aβ which can then aggregate into insoluble deposit such as diffuse and neuritic plaques.

The most compelling evidence supporting the amyloid hypothesis comes from genetic studies of autosomal dominant forms of AD (for a review see Hardy and Selkoe[200]). All of the known causative mutations for AD in the *APP* gene cluster at or near sites normally cleaved by alpha, beta, and gamma secretases. These *APP* gene mutations lead to increased generation of Aβ by favoring proteolytic processing of APP by beta or gamma secretase. *Presenilin 1* and *presenilin 2* mutations enhance processing of APP to form amyloidogenic Aβ through direct effects on gamma secretase. Each of these rare mutations is associated with high Aβ production and lead to early-onset AD. The susceptibility factor, *ApoE*, appears also to promote Aβ deposition and its conversion to a fibrillary form that results in neuritic plaques. Another susceptibility locus for AD recently has been reported on chromosome 10 and also is associated with high plasma levels of $A\beta_{1-42}$. Multiple lines of evidence support the critical role of amyloid in the pathogenesis of AD and provide rationale for the prevention of accumulation and deposition of amyloid as a therapeutic target.[200]

If the amyloid hypothesis indeed is relevant to AD, it is conceivable that disease-modifying approaches will substantially improve the ability to provide meaningful treatment of AD, or even to prevent its occurrence. The amyloid hypothesis is the basis for at least six broad therapeutic strategies, including neuroprotection, secretase inhibition, amyloid vaccination, anti-inflammatory treatments, cholesterol reduction, and chelation therapy.

Secretase inhibitors

APP processing via the alternative pathway may be an integral step in the production of insoluble amyloid found prominently in plaques. Drugs that block the alternative processing of APP by inhibiting beta- and gamma-secretase activity[203] are being developed. These agents are postulated to reduce the accumulation and deposition of Aβ. Clinical trials are currently underway on gamma-secretase inhibitors. The development of beta-secretase inhibitors has been hindered by difficulties in identifying small molecules capable of fitting the large active site of beta secretase (an aspartyl protease) while still maintaining an ability to cross the blood–brain barrier.

Amyloid vaccine

Immunization strategies are the subject of intense research as a possible amyloid-lowering strategy. Interest in this technique arose after immunization strategies were employed in mice. In these initial studies, mice bred to express AD pathology (*APP* transgenic mice) generated an immune response that prevented deposition and promoted microglial clearance of cerebral Aβ plaques after Aβ immunization.[204–206] Additional benefits in learning and memory were observed.

In 2001, the strategy was tested in a phase-2 vaccination trial in 375 individuals with AD. The trial was halted in 2002 when 15 of the treated subjects developed symptomatic brain inflammation (meningoencephalitis). One subject has since died, and neuropathological evaluation revealed extensive cortical areas with little plaque pathology despite the presence of neurofibrillary tangles. Additionally, there were findings consistent with a T-lymphocyte menigoencephalitis, suggesting an active immune response to the antibody that cleared the amyloid plaques.[207] In a separate retrospective evaluation,[208] a subset of individuals ($n = 19$) antibodies appeared to have slower cognitive decline than those without antibodies ($n = 9$). Despite a prohibitively large number of adverse events, the data generated in this trial suggest that the immune response may be stimulated to reduce amyloid plaques in the brain of individuals with AD.

The concept has already provided the basis for other promising and novel techniques such as passive immunization, selective targeting of fragments of amyloid, or simultaneous administration of anti-inflammatory agents. Additionally, it has been observed that antibodies need not enter the central nervous system to reduce brain amyloid. Instead, the creation of an Aβ-concentration gradient between brain and blood may act as a sink to alter the brain-plasma equilibrium, leading to reductions in brain Aβ burden.[209] These, and other, immunization techniques may someday be useful in the treatment of AD.

Potential biomarkers

Using contemporary diagnostic criteria, AD diagnoses in specialized centers are accurate 80–90% of the time. The clinical diagnosis of AD is currently made after careful medical history and neurological examination. Laboratory studies and brain imaging are important in excluding underlying metabolic or structural etiologies. The ability to detect the presence of disease using a simple blood, cerebrospinal fluid, or neuroimaging test would be very useful in the early diagnosis of disease and in monitoring disease progression. Thus, the identification of AD biomarkers is the focus of intense research (Table 6.1).

The Reagan Institute of the Alzheimer's Association and the National Institute of Aging convened a working group in 1997 to examine further the issue of biomarkers in AD.[210] Their statement outlined the characteristics of a model biomarker. Ideally, a biomarker should detect a fundamental feature of AD neuropathology and should be validated using neuropathologically confirmed AD cases. A biomarker should be precise in that it should detect AD early in its course and distinguish it from other dementias. The sensitivity and specificity of an AD biomarker should be at least 80%, with a positive predictive value approaching 90%. Furthermore, a clinically useful biomarker should be reliable, non-invasive, simple to perform, and inexpensive.

Several candidate biomarkers for AD and other dementias are under investigation. These proposed diagnostic tests will need to be highly sensitive and specific to prove better than already highly accurate clinical methods. No single test, however, has yet demonstrated a better diagnostic sensitivity and specificity than an evaluation by an experienced clinician, and currently there is insufficient evidence to recommend cerebrospinal fluid (CSF) or

TABLE 6.1 Putative biomarkers

CSF
- Beta-amyloid
- Tau
- Sulfatide
- Markers of inflammation
  - Interleukin (IL) 6, IL-1B, tumor necrosis factor, α_1-antichymortrypsin, haptoglobin
- Markers of oxidative stress
  - 4-hydroxynonenal, F2-isoprostanes, F4-neuroprotanes, 8-hydrodeoxyguanine, 3-nitrotyrosine

Serum
- Beta-amyloid

Neuroimaging
- MRI
  - Hippocampal volume
  - Whole brain volume
  - Rates of atrophy (whole brain, hippocampal)
- Functional Imaging
  - Positron emission tomography (PET)
  - Single photon computed tomography (SPECT)
  - Functional MRI
- Amyloid labeling

Genetic Testing
- Amyloid precursor protein
- *Presenelin 1* and *Presenelin 2*
- *Apolipoprotein E*

plasma biomarkers, genetic testing, or functional imaging in the diagnosis of AD (Table 6.1).

CSF biomarkers

Several potential CSF markers of AD have been investigated and include forms of beta-amyloid (Aβ), tau, and various markers of oxidative stress and inflammation. Despite all the promising results,

CSF markers are not more accurate than clinical diagnosis alone and should not be routinely assessed in patients with cognitive impairment.

CSF beta-amyloid (Aβ)

The levels of CSF Aβ have been postulated to reflect the central pathogenic process of senile plaques. Aβ proteins are derived from proteolytic processing of the amyloid precursor protein (APP) which primarily yields two Aβ proteins of different length: $A\beta_{1-42}$ and $A\beta_{1-40}$. $A\beta_{1-40}$ tends to be soluble and is present in high concentrations in the brain, while $A\beta_{1-42}$ is highly amyloidogenic, insoluble and is an initial component of senile plaques.

Multiple studies have reported lower CSF $A\beta_{1-42}$ levels in individuals with AD compared with non-demented controls. CSF levels of $A\beta_{1-42}$ may represent increased incorporation of the CSF $A\beta_{1-42}$ into amyloid plaques,[211–213] with less remaining in the CSF, resulting in lower levels in AD subjects. The concentration of $A\beta_{1-40}$ is generally unchanged. Initial studies have demonstrated that CSF Aβ levels can distinguish AD subjects from controls with moderate sensitivities (78–92%) and specificities (81–83%).[214–216]

CSF tau

The main protein component of neurofibrillary tangles (NFTs) is the microtubule-associated protein tau. In healthy neurons, tau stabilizes axonal microtubules. In AD, tau becomes abnormally hyperphosphorylated, resulting in its dissociation from micro-tubules and self-assembly into paired helical filaments. This process appears to be involved in the formation of the neurofibrillary tangle. The level of tau in CSF has been suggested to reflect neuronal and axonal degeneration and the formation of NFTs.

CSF tau has been shown to be significantly elevated in patients with AD compared with controls. CSF tau distinguished AD patients from controls, with a sensitivity of 80–97% and a specificity of 86–95%.[217] The diagnostic yield may improve with concomitant measurement of CSF tau and Aβ.[212,216] Combined analysis of CSF Aβ$_{1-42}$ and tau levels has been used to discriminate AD and control subjects in a clinical setting with 90% sensitivity and 80% specificity.[212] In a community-based population sample, combined analysis of Aβ$_{1-42}$ and tau yielded 94% sensitivity for detecting probable AD, 88% for possible AD, and 75% for mild cognitive impairment.[214] Specificity was high in differentiating non-demented and psychiatric diagnoses. Before CSF measures of tau and Aβ$_{1-42}$ can be utilized in a clinical setting, further prospective studies with neuropathological assessment will be necessary to verify these findings (Figure 6.3).

CSF sulfatide

Sulfatides are sulfated galactocerebrosides that mediate diverse biological processes. Sulfatides (ST) are synthesized by oligodendrocytes in the CNS (central nervous system) and comprise 5% of myelin. In the brains of those in the earliest stages of AD,

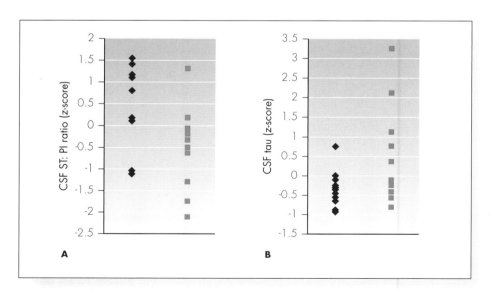

FIGURE 6.3 (A) CSF sulfatide: phosphatidylinositol ratio; **(B)** CSF tau. CSF measures, such as tau and sulfatide, reveal group mean differences between AD (grey) and non-demented controls. The overlap between groups, however, is substantial and limits their clinical utility. Combinations of tests may better discriminate the earliest changes of AD from non-demented aging.

there is a 58% decrease in white-matter sulfatide and a 93% decrease in gray-matter sulfatide. ST levels are markedly reduced in the brains of early AD subjects at autopsy[218,219] and in the CSF of living subjects in the earliest clinical stages of AD.[220] CSF ST is speculated to reflect axonal damage or degeneration.[220,221]

Han *et al.*[220] studied the CSF from 20 individuals with very mild dementia and found a 40% decline in CSF sulfatide compared with non-demented controls. The ability of sulfatide to discriminate the very mildly demented from non-demented was compared with amyloid beta and tau measures in the same individuals. The overlap between the very mildly demented and non-demented was very high using amyloid beta and tau, while sulfatide had much better discrimination (90% sensitivity and 100% specificity). These findings need validation in larger samples and other neurodegenerative dementia before sulfatide can be considered a viable clinical bio-marker.

CSF markers of inflammation

Mediators of inflammation have been found in amyloid plaques and may play a role in the pathogenesis of AD. Epidemiological studies provide evidence that the use of anti-inflammatory drugs may reduce the prevalence of dementia, additional evidence that inflammation is involved in the pathogenesis of AD. Elevated levels of IL-1β, IL-6, tumor necrosis factor, α_1-antichymortrypsin, and haptoglobin have been reported in the CSF and serum of AD patients, although these results have not been uniformly replicated.[223] More research is needed to establish the usefulness of inflammatory markers in differentiating AD from normal controls.

CSF markers of oxidative stress

There is increasing evidence to support the role of oxidative stress in neurodegenerative disorders. Markers of oxidative stress are present in neurofibrillary tangles and senile plaques. Oxidative damage has been demonstrated in the brains of AD subjects. Increased levels of protein oxidation and markers of lipid peroxidation such as

4-hydroxynonenal, F2-isoprostanes, and F4-neuroprostanes have been demonstrated in brain tissue and CSF. Quantification of F2-isoprostanes has emerged as an accurate approach for the assessment of oxidative damage *in vivo*.[223] Attack of DNA by reactive oxygen species leads to hydroxylation of DNA and generation of 8-hydrodeoxyguanine, which is elevated in the cerebral cortex of AD patients compared with controls.[224] An early marker of oxidative stress may be 3-nitrotyrosine in neurodegenerative disorders, and it has been reported to be elevated in the CSF of patients with AD, Parkinson's disease, and amyotrophic lateral sclerosis.

Serum biomarkers

A simple blood test would be the ideal method for detecting the presence of AD. A number of potential peripheral biomarkers have been investigated, but further research is necessary before their potential clinical applicability can be explored.

Plasma $A\beta$ assays have been studied, but with exception of some reports of increased $A\beta_{1-42}$ levels in individuals with causative AD mutations, the results have been equivocal. In a cross-sectional study of plasma $A\beta$ levels in patients with AD, MCI, Parkinson's disease, and non-demented aging, the strongest determinant of $A\beta$ levels in each group was age alone.[225] Plasma levels of $A\beta_{1-42}$ are unlikely to be of clinical utility by themselves. A promising strategy involves facilitating the CNS clearance of $A\beta$ using $A\beta$ antibodies. DeMattos et al.[226] intravenously administered a monoclonal $A\beta$ antibody (m266) to *APP* transgenic mice and found a rapid and marked increase in plasma $A\beta_{1-40}$ and $A\beta_{1-42}$ within 5 min of administration. The increase in $A\beta$ levels was correlated with the level of hippocampal $A\beta$ burden. Using this technique, the presence of "high" and "low" plaque burden in the brains of affected, living mice could be predicted. The administration of the m266 $A\beta$ antibody in the peripheral circulation thus directly facilitated $A\beta$ efflux from the brain, acting as a "peripheral sink". The investigators concluded that brain $A\beta$ is dynamically processed and that modifications of its processing may be useful in the diagnosis and treatment of AD.

Structural imaging

Currently, the major role of structural neuroimaging (CT and MRI) is in excluding potentially dementing disorders. A number of techniques are being explored in an attempt to identify neuroimaging findings that may be included to support the diagnosis of AD. The major thrust has been in identifying neuroanatomic changes, such as atrophy, that may predict cognitive decline related to AD. Neuroanatomic changes have been consistently linked with primary brain pathology.[86] Substantial evidence exists to the effect that MRI volumetrics are a valid biomarker for AD pathological progression, indirectly detecting cell loss and correlating with AD neuropathological burden.[86–88] Atrophy, however, is associated to some degree with non-demented aging, and difficulty arises in distinguishing "pathological" atrophy from "normal" atrophy (Figure 6.4).

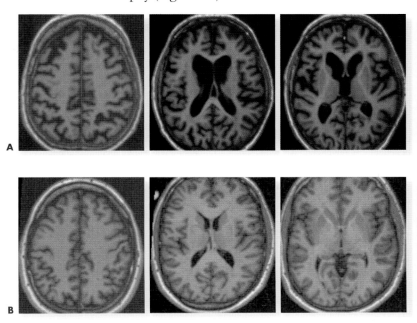

FIGURE 6.4 Global atrophy is apparent in the brain of a 90 year old nondemented man **(A)**. The ventricles are significantly enlarged with prominent sulci. For comparison, a 39 year old nondemented man **(B)** at corresponding levels shows smaller ventricles, fuller white matter, and less prominent sulci. Courtesy of Randy L. Buckner.

Great emphasis has been placed on measurements of the medial temporal lobe as clinically useful markers of neurodegeneration. Medial temporal lobe volume loss is seen in AD and in MCI patients. Du *et al.* found reduced volumes in both MCI and AD subjects compared with non-demented controls. The MCI group had a 13% reduction in the entorhinal cortex and 11% reduction of the hippocampus. AD subjects were more severely affected, with 39% reduction of entorhinal cortex and 27% reduction of the hippocampus. Jack et al.[79] followed 80 MCI subjects longitudinally and found that baseline hippocampal volume was predictive of progression to further stages of impairment (Figure 6.5).

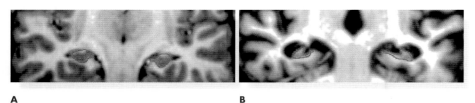

A   B

FIGURE 6.5 Hippocampal volumes are reduced in the earliest stages of AD compared to nondemented controls. In this figure, the hippocampi of an 86 year old woman with Alzheimer disease show large difference in size compared to a young, health male. (Courtesy of Denise Head and Randy L. Buckner)

Measurements of the medial temporal lobe may prove to be clinically useful markers of AD, although atrophy is not disease specific. Serial measurements may prove to be useful in monitoring disease progression, although more work is necessary before these measures can be widely employed or recommended in the evaluation of patients with cognitive decline.

Functional neuroimaging

Functional imaging studies using PET (positron emission tomography), SPECT (single-photon emission computed tomography (SPECT), and fMRI (functional magnetic resonance imaging) have sought to identify a physiological or neuroanatomic signature corresponding to the clinical symptoms of AD. At this point, no data support the widespread use of functional neuroimaging for routine diagnosis.

PET and SPECT

PET and SPECT are nuclear medicine techniques that involve injection and visualization of a radiolabeled substance in the brain to infer information about neural activity. These techniques are based on the premise that the brain absorbs the radiolabeled substances in proportion to the metabolic demands of the tissue.

PET uses radiotracers that emit positrons, most commonly $[^{18}F]$ deoxyglucose (FDG), a glucose analog labeled with ^{18}fluorine. This analog is taken up by the brain and metabolized. SPECT uses technetium-labeled substances that are taken up by the brain in proportion to blood flow but do not readily exit the brain. PET image acquisition occurs just after the radiotracer is administered and imaging reflects the radiotracer's metabolism. SPECT image acquisition can occur anytime within several hours after injection. The image represents the cerebral state during the several minutes that the tracer was absorbed by the brain. SPECT costs substantially less and has greater availability given the wide use of gamma cameras in nuclear cardiology.

PET and SPECT studies have demonstrated functional changes in the brains of AD subjects. AD-associated hypometabolism in posterior cortical regions has been reported consistently and has been proposed as an early diagnostic marker of AD.[90,91]

Most studies have reported temporoparietal abnormalities early in the course of the disease, with frontal abnormalities developing later.[227] The posterior regions are hypothesized to be involved early in the disease process given the dense interconnections with medial temporal regions;[228] these areas are involved in memory processing and are among the earliest and most prominent sites of AD pathology.[229] Lesions (in animals and humans) in the entorhinal cortex and the perirhinal cortex result in decreased posterior cingulate metabolism similar that seen in AD.[230–234] Thus, posterior cortical regions, in particular the posterior cingulate and the precuneus, appear to be part of the memory system and AD-related hypometabolism may therefore reflect memory impairment[235–238] (Figure 6.6).

In patients with cognitive impairment judged not to be demented, SPECT demonstrated temporoparietal hypoperfusion that was intermediate between that found in normal controls and in patients with AD.[92] In another SPECT study[93], questionable AD patients who later converted to AD had reduced perfusion of the hippocampus and posterior cingulate when compared with those who did not decline. De Leon *et al.*[90] followed normal elderly subjects and found that metabolic reductions in the entorhinal cortex accurately predicted the "conversion" from normal to MCI with entorhinal cortical changes occurring in advance of symptomatic decline.

Metabolic deficits have been reported in unaffected individuals at high risk of the development of dementia. Early metabolic deficits in the temporoparietal region and the posterior cingulate cortex have been reported in asymptomatic individuals at risk for familial AD.[239] Temporoparietal metabolic deficits were also apparent in cognitively normal subjects at risk for AD by being homozygous for the *ApoE4* allele.[240]

Although SPECT and PET may be useful in differentiating AD from other non-AD forms of dementia (e.g. frontotemporal dementia), further prospective studies are necessary to determine the value of functional imaging and to address what additional value a SPECT and PET scan provides to the already accurate clinical diagnosis.

Functional MRI (fMRI)

Functional MRI (fMRI) is a powerful technique for measuring the brain activity of subjects while performing memory or cognitive tasks. Most fMRI studies utilize the changes in blood flow that accompany increased neural activity. Increases in blood oxygen content can be imaged with MRI (this is called the blood oxygen level dependent (BOLD) mechanism) and then used as an indirect measure of neural activity.

Non-demented individuals at high risk for developing AD (by virtue of being *APOE4* allele carriers) were studied using fMRI, and

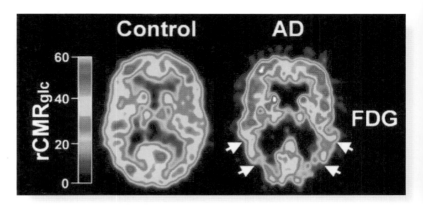

FIGURE 6.6 Positron emission tomogrophy (PET) images from a non-demented control and an individual with AD. Typical findings include reduced metabolism in the temporoparietal cortices as indicated by lower uptake of 18F-fluorodeoxyglucose (FDG). rCMRglc indicates cerebral glucose metabolic rate. Reprinted with permission of John Wiley & Sons, Inc.[246]

demonstrated a different pattern of brain activation than *APOE3* homozygotes.[241] The magnitude and extent of brain activation during memory tasks was greater in those at risk of AD, suggesting additional cognitive work was needed in these subjects to accomplish successfully the cognitive task. Longitudinal assessment of these individuals over 2 years revealed that the degree of base-line brain activation correlated with the degree of decline in memory. The authors concluded that patterns of brain activation differed depending on the genetic risk of AD and may predict a subsequent decline in memory. In another study of individuals at high risk of AD, Smith *et al.*[242] found significantly reduced activation in temporal regions during naming and letter-fluency tasks despite normal performance on these tasks (Figure 6.7).

Lustig *et al.*[243] investigated the dynamic activity profiles of the posterior cingulate cortex in young, older non-demented , and early-stage AD subjects. Both quantitative and qualitative differences in the posterior cingulate region were observed in all groups, with early-stage AD subjects demonstrating a marked positive activation in this area. This increased posterior cingulate activity in AD has

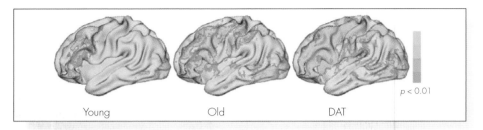

FIGURE 6.7 Statistical activation maps showing fMRI measurements of brain activity in young adults (YNG), nondemented older adults (OLD, CDR = 0), and older adults in the early stages of dementia of the Alzheimer type (DAT, CDR = 0.5 or 1). Activations are projected onto a slightly inflated representation of and were obtained during a simple word classification task (living/nonliving) that promotes memory for words. Note that all three groups show strong activation in regions of left frontal cortex. (Courtesy of Cindy Lustig and Randy L. Buckner).

been postulated to represent a response to AD neuropathological changes in the medial temporal lobe, as suggested by the medial temporal lobe's major projection fibers to the posterior cingulate and the resulting hypometabolism of the posterior cingulate when these fibers are disrupted.[228,230–233]

Functional changes may occur before substantial neuronal loss has occurred and may serve as a preclinical marker for AD. fMRI is a powerful tool for characterizing age-related changes in functional anatomy that may perhaps provide functional-anatomic markers predictive of cognitive decline associated with AD.

Imaging amyloid

The molecular imaging of amyloid deposits has promise as a potential biomarker for AD and possibly may allow the identification of individuals who are still in the presymptomatic stages of the illness. Radioligands have been developed that cross the blood–brain barrier and bind specifically to Aβ aggregates in sufficient amounts to be imaged by PET.[244,245]

In a proof-of-concept PET study, a benzothiole amyloid agent, also known as Pittsburgh compound-B (PIB), resulted in significantly higher standardized uptake values in 16 AD patients compared with 6 elderly control subjects in regions known to have extensive amyloid deposition.[246] Preferential retention of PIB in frontal and temporoparietal cortex discriminated between most mild AD individuals and control subjects. These initial results suggest that PET imaging with amyloid tracer may quantify cerebral amyloid in living humans (Figure 6.8).

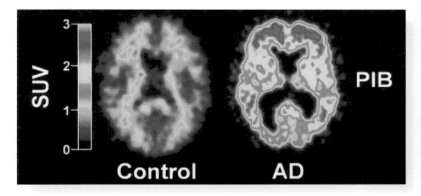

FIGURE 6.8 Amyloid imaging. The Pittsburgh Compond B (PIB) uptake is significantly increased in the individual with Alzheimer's disease versus the control as indicated by higher standardized uptake values (SUV) throughout the cortex. Reprinted with permission of John Wiley & Sons, Inc.[246]

As research using these compounds progresses, data is emerging to suggest that some nondemented individuals with no clinical symptoms of dementia have increased retention of the amyloid-labeling agent.[10] In a study including 41 nondemented subjects age 20–86, there were four individuals with retention of the PIB compound that was comparable to the values seen in individuals with AD. This has led to the hypothesis that amyloid imaging may be sensitive for the detection of AD pathology prior to the onset of symptoms. Longitudinal studies are necessary to determine if these individuals will develop the clinical syndrome of AD and to further define the role of molecular imaging methods in identifying individuals with preclinical AD.

Genetic testing

Genetic factors clearly play a role in the development of AD. Single-gene defects probably account for less than 1% of all AD cases. Most cases of AD are likely a result of both genetic and environmental risk factors. The genetic complexity and heterogeneity of AD, therefore limits the predictive value of genetic tests.

Early-onset familial AD

Early-onset AD – occurring before 60 years of age – accounts for roughly 5% of AD cases. Early-onset AD is often characterized by autosomal dominant inheritance with virtually 100% penetration. Three gene defects are known to cause early-onset familial AD: the amyloid precursor protein gene (*APP*), *presenilin 1 (PS-1)*, and *presenilin 2 (PS-2)*.

The predictive value of genetic tests in early-onset AD has not been formally tested. The appeal for diagnostic tests is high, and the marketing of AD genetic tests is growing. Genetic testing is a complex issue involving multiple personal and social issues that must be taken into account prior to testing. For instance, roughly 40% of early-onset AD families will not have an identifiable mutation given the allelic heterogeneity. Thus, a negative test result is non-diagnostic. Positive identification of a mutation has ramifications for the patient's extended family and raises confidentiality issues. Genetic testing should not be performed routinely, but should proceed only in the context of fully informed consent, pre- and post-testing genetic counseling, and careful protection of confidentiality.

Amyloid precursor protein

The amyloid precursor protein (*APP*) gene on chromosome 21 was the first gene to be genetically linked to familial AD. The age of onset of AD in individuals with an *APP* mutation ranges from 39 to 67 years. Mutations of APP account for only 2–3% of the early-onset familial cases.

Most of the *APP* mutations cluster at or near sites within *APP* that are normally cleaved by the α-, β-, and γ-secretases. The mutations appear to facilitate the formation of Aβ by promoting APP processing with the β-, and γ-secretases. *APP* mutations within the Aβ site appear to increase the self-aggregation of Aβ into fibrils. Incidentally, mice with *APP* mutations produce numerous amyloid plaques, but are generally without significant neurofibrillary tangles and synaptic loss.

Presenilin genes

The presenilins are believed to be part of the γ-secretase complex, and mutations in these genes appear to enhance the processing of APP to form amyloidogenic Aβ. *Presenilin 1 (PS-1)* was identified in 1995 on chromosome 14. More than 50 different AD mutations in more than 80 families have been identified in *PS-1*, accounting for roughly 30–40% of early-onset AD. The vast majority of AD in *PS-1* mutation carriers have an onset of disease under the age of 50 years.

The *PS-2* gene was isolated on chromosome 1, based on its extensive genetic homology to *PS-1*. It was discovered as the causative mutation of AD in a group of related families from the Volga River region in Russia. *PS-2* has been found to contain only two different mutations. The mean age of onset of AD in *PS-2* carriers is 52 years old; however, the range of ages is quite broad, varying in onset from 40–85 years (Table 6.2).

TABLE 6.2 Alzheimer's disease genes and amyloid-beta

Chromosome	Gene defect	Dementia onset age	Aβ phenotype
21	*APP* mutations	50s	Increased total Aβ and $A\beta_{1-42}$
19	*Apolipoprotein E4 polymorphism*	60s+	Increased Aβ deposits
14	*Presenilin 1*	40s and 50s	Increased $A\beta_{1-42}$
1	*Presenilin 2*	50s	Increased $A\beta_{1-42}$

Late-onset AD

Late-onset AD is by far the most common form of AD. Late-onset AD is much more complex than early-onset forms of AD and clearly involves both genetics and the environment. Difficulties in unraveling the genetics of late-onset AD arise for several reasons. The baseline rate of AD is high with aging, and therefore some familial clustering may be chance alone. As AD occurs late in life, many individuals do not survive to manifest AD, making assessment of the mode of inheritance difficult. A number of genes and gene linkages have been reported to be associated with AD, but the *ApoE* gene is the only established genetic risk factor.

Apolipoprotein E

Apolipoprotein E (*ApoE*) is the only recognized genetic risk factor for late-onset AD, the most common form of AD. *ApoE* is a genetic polymorphism (i.e. it has common variations) that exist as three major alleles: *E2*, *E3*, and *E4* on chromosome 19. Multiple studies have established that carrying an *E4* allele increases the risk for AD in a dose-dependent manner (two alleles confer a higher risk than one) and is associated with an earlier age at onset of the disease.[247] In contrast, the presence of an *E2* allele confers protection against AD. *ApoE* probably modifies the expression of AD through interactions with Aβ that increase the deposition of amyloid in plaques.

Testing for the presence of *ApoE4* is not necessary in diagnosing AD, and routine assessment is not justified. The presence of *ApoE4* slightly increases the positive predictive value of a clinical diagnosis of AD (from 90% to 94%) while the absence of *ApoE4* increases the negative predictive value (from 64% to 72%).[248] Roughly 50% of individuals with AD carry one or more *ApoE4* alleles, However, carrying an *ApoE4* allele does not mean the individual inevitably will develop AD, as only approximately 50% of *ApoE* carriers will develop the disease. Routine *ApoE* testing has no role in the routine diagnosis of AD and is not currently recommended.

Case studies

The following case studies are examples drawn from our database of longitudinally non-demented and demented older adults. They are provided in an effort to encapsulate many of the ideas regarding MCI (mild cognitive impairment) and early AD (Alzheimer's disease) presented in this text. The first case demonstrates that the diagnosis of AD can be made accurately in the setting of MCI. Despite functioning at a high level and meeting criteria for MCI, the patient demonstrated acquired cognitive impairments that interfered, albeit subtly, with function in daily activities and thus met criteria for dementia. The second case demonstrates that the diagnosis of early AD can be made before psychometric tests detect decline and even before an individual meets criteria for MCI. The third case demonstrates difficulties in making the diagnosis, given the common nature of memory complaints with age. A clinician must weigh carefully the factors that contribute to memory complaints and diligently probe for characteristic features of AD.

Case report 1: MCI as early-stage Alzheimer's disease

A retired university professor with a doctorate in metallurgy was first evaluated at 78 years of age; his wife (to whom he had been married for 55 years) served as the collateral source. He was in excellent health ("skin cancers" had been excised the previous year), and he took no prescription medications (he used vitamin E 800 IU daily throughout his participation). There was no history of depression, past or present. His wife reported an 18-month history of gradually progressive "short-term memory loss" in her husband. He was repetitive, asking the same question she had already answered. He misplaced important documents, and his home office was uncharacteristically cluttered. He now experienced some difficulty in balancing the checkbook and made a dubious large investment without his wife's approval. However, he was involved productively in many activities, including tutoring elementary-school students, teaching metallurgy to Elder Hostel participants, and serving on church committees. He drove without any problems, played word games and cards, and was fully independent in self-care. The subject conceded that "I forget somethings sometimes" but did not consider this to be a problem. He performed all brief cognitive tests of recall, orientation, calculations, and clock drawing without difficulty, but forgot important details of recent events in which he had participated (e.g. attending a major-league baseball game with friends). He weighed 85 kg (187 lb); the neurological examination was unremarkable.

Based on his wife's subjective report of subtle, but definite, cognitive decline involving memory and executive function (judgment and problem solving) and his inability to recall recent personal events, he was staged as very mild dementia (CDR 0.5); the diagnosis was Alzheimer's disease (AD). Donepezil was initiated, but self-terminated after a few weeks because of "bad dreams".

The subject's annual assessment at the age of 79 years yielded a history and findings that were very similar to his baseline evaluation. He now needed more direction from his wife to reach destinations when driving, and she had assumed more responsibility for the household finances. He also needed prompting to shave. He again was rated CDR 0.5, with a diagnosis of AD. At his third assessment (age 80 years), his wife reported that he repeated the same question "over and over". He missed meetings because he was confused as to the date and time. He forgot to relay telephone messages to his wife. However, he correctly calculated tips "in his head" at restaurants, shopped independently for needs, drove without accident, maintained his yard and garden, and continued to play games without obvious impairment. Although there was no depression, his wife commented that he had "less initiative". He remained physically healthy without prescription medications. He self-reported his memory as "not unusual"; brief cognitive-test performance was good, except that he was impaired in recalling recent personal events. The diagnosis remained AD at the CDR 0.5 stage. He was enrolled in a double-blind, placebo-controlled clinical trial of an anti-inflammatory agent to evaluate possible cognitive benefits. Head computed tomography obtained as part of his trial participation suggested two small cerebellar hemispheric infarctions but otherwise was unremarkable.

There were no major changes at his next annual assessment at the age of 81 years. He recently had presented a report on Stonehenge to the men's group at his church; although the report went well, he required an unusually long time to prepare it. He now required prompting to shower daily. He did well on most brief cognitive tests, but for the first time had difficulty recalling a five-item memory phrase. He again weighed 85 kg (187 lb). The diagnosis (AD) and stage (CDR 0.5) remained as before.

At the age of 82 years, he was becoming lost when driving alone outside his neighborhood and had relinquished household finances to his wife. He did not recall personal events of even the preceding week. He now was using galantamine for symptomatic treatment of AD. He was disoriented regarding both the month and the year; however, he still performed simple calculations correctly. He was rated CDR 1 (mild dementia) for the first time. A formal driving evaluation found his skills to be "intact", but noted that he would be at risk of becoming lost in unfamiliar areas. At the age of 83 years, he remained on galantamine. His wife reported that he continued to drive and attend the men's club at his church. However, he forgot conversations quickly, needed prompting to work in the yard, and had his clothes "set out" for him by his wife. He again was disoriented regarding both the month and the year and recalled none of the five-item memory phrase; however, he still did simple calculations correctly. The CDR remained 1.

His most recent assessment was at the age of 84 years. He again weighed 85 kg (187 lb) and remained in excellent physical health. His only prescription medication was galantamine (4 mg twice daily); additional drugs included vitamin E (800 IU daily) and ginkgo biloba.

His wife reported that his memory continued to deteriorate. Six months earlier, he failed to recognize his destination when driving, inadvertently entered an interstate highway and drove for several hours into another state before running out of fuel. The State's Highway Patrol helped his wife locate him and bring him home. He required supervision at home for even simple chores, such as feeding the dog. His performance on brief cognitive tests was comparable with that of the previous year. However, he incorrectly thought his age was "85", did not know how long he had been married, and no longer remembered his occupation. He stated that he retired "in 1932".

Comment

This intelligent, highly educated man developed early symptoms of dementia at approximately 76 years of age. Cognitive impairment, albeit very mild, was reported 2 years later by his wife for memory (e.g. frequent repetition; misplacement of items) and judgment and problem solving (e.g. difficulty balancing the checkbook; inappropriate investment). He still functioned at a high level in many activities in the community and at home. Brief cognitive tests did not show impairment. However, deficits were apparent on a more "face-valid" test of memory (recall of recent autobiographical events). His neuropsychological test performance (Table 7.1) met

TABLE 7.1 Case report 1: Cognitive test performance

Assessment	Age (years)	WMS Logical memory (9±2)	Digit span- backwards (5±1)	Mini-mental state exam (28.9±1.3)	Short Blessed test (1.3±2.1)	CDR	Clinical diagnosis
1	78	5.5	5	29	2	0.5	AD
2	79	3.5	4	26	8	0.5	AD
3	80	3.5	5	27	2	0.5	AD
4	81	4.0	6	26	6	0.5	AD
5	82	3.5	6	22	8	1	AD
6	83	1.0	4	24	18	1	AD
7	84	3.5	6	22	13	1	AD

CDR = clinical dementia rating (0 = no dementia, 0.5 = very mild dementia, 1 = mild dementia); AD = Alzheimer's disease; WMS = Wechsler memory scale; Mean scores of non-demented subjects in the same study as this individual are shown in parentheses for each measure. Higher scores indicate better performance for all measures except the short Blessed test, where lower scores are better.

criteria for MCI: objective deficit in an episodic memory measure (logical memory) and "generally preserved" cognitive performance otherwise (MMSE score = 29). The history (primarily the subjective report from his wife) indicated an acquired impairment in memory and in at least one other cognitive domain that was just beginning to interfere with his conduct of accustomed activities (e.g. household finances). That is, he met clinical criteria for dementia of the Alzheimer type at its earliest symptomatic stages with highly characteristic features ("short-term memory loss", frequent repetition, misplacement of items). Figure 7.1 plots psychometric factor score and CDR against time of testing for this patient.

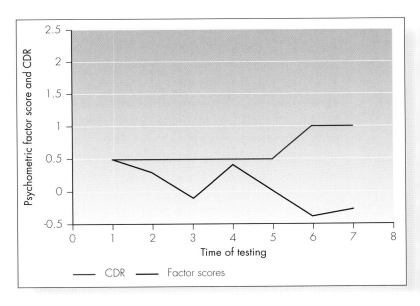

FIGURE 7.1 Case study 1: Longitudinal cognitive performance and dementia severity.

A less comprehensive collateral-source interview (or a less observant informant) or reliance on neuropsychological test performance, rather than on the subjective information, almost certainly would have resulted in a diagnosis of "MCI, insufficient to meet criteria for dementia". However, the original diagnosis of very mild AD was supported by the subsequent clinical, cognitive, and functional decline experienced by this individual.

Case report 2: Diagnosis of dementia prior to impairment sufficient for MCI

At 69 years of age, a right-handed widowed retired electrical engineer (college graduate) was enrolled in a longitudinal study of memory and aging. There was no family history of dementia. Other than laminectomy for left sciatica 3 years earlier, he enjoyed excellent health and took no prescription medications. He had no children and lived independently. A close friend served as collateral source. The friend reported that his money and thinking abilities were excellent; he had "the best memory of anyone". He was a volunteer teacher for a community college, led book discussion groups at his church, and regularly played bridge, chess, and other games. He enjoyed attending movies with friends and patronized the theater. He golfed, bowled, and exercised daily. He did his own income-tax preparations and assisted friends with theirs. He drove an automobile, shopped, and maintained his apartment without problems. There was no indication of depression or personality change. The subject himself had no complaints regarding memory and thinking. He did well on all brief clinical measures of memory, orientation, calculation, and clock drawing. The neurological examination was unremarkable. He was enrolled as a non-demented control participant with CDR = 0. All subsequent annual assessments through to the age of 77 years yielded identical clinical information and CDR 0 scores.

Between the ages of 77 and 84 years, the subject had a prostatectomy, was briefly hospitalized with pneumonia, had basal cell cancers excised from the face, and was treated as an outpatient for bleeding diverticula. However, he still required no routine prescription drugs. His neurological status remained normal, his weight remained at about 70 kg (154 lbs), and there was no evidence of depression.

At the age of 78 years, for the first time the subject self-reported a memory problem that was "hard to pinpoint". He complained about difficulty in recalling names of persons he knew well but acknowledged that the names came to him later. He reported being forgetful and "not as sharp mentally". Increasing memory complaints from the subject characterized all subsequent clinical assessments through to the age of 90 years. At the age of 78 years, his friend reported that he now occasionally lost to her at card games, forgot "trivial" details, and seemed to be "slowing down" mentally, but she did not consider these memory and thinking changes to represent a "problem"; nor did they interfere with his performance of accustomed activities (he remained as engaged as before). His performance on the brief clinical measures remained completely normal.

At the age of 81 years, his friend noticed that he occasionally forgot movies they had seen together, but considered these lapses "normal for age". He still was as active as usual, continuing as leader of the book club and playing golf, cards, and chess. However, he uncharacteristically had made errors in helping a friend prepare her tax return. His performance on the brief clinical measures again was intact, and he still was judged to be non-demented. At the age of 83 years, the friend noted that he now erred in card playing and occasionally repeated questions or statements. At 84 years of age, there were further changes. He had misplaced his passport on a European trip, made errors in his tax return, grasped fewer details of books he had read, and had "less clear reasoning". He forgot conversations and repeated stories. However, he remained leader of his book club, drove without difficulty, and lived independently. The subject reported that his memory was "deteriorating" and that he was "slower" to solve puzzles. There was no depression. His brief clinical cognitive performance showed no errors. Based on the subjective reports of decline in memory and reasoning (e.g. errors on tax returns), for the first time he was considered to be very mildly demented at the CDR 0.5 stage, and was diagnosed with incipient Alzheimer's disease (AD) at the age of 84 years.

At his next two annual assessments, in spite of similar reports of subtle cognitive change from both the collateral source and the subject, his intact cognitive performances on the clinical measures persuaded raters that he was CDR 0. By the age of 87 years, however, he again was rated CDR 0.5 (diagnosed with uncertain dementia). He had declined physically; he had sustained a rib fracture in a fall and also was evaluated for diarrhea. He weighed 65 kg (143 lbs). He had begun using hearing aids. He was considered to be depressed, based on symptoms such as loss of energy, loss of interest, and thoughts of death, and referred to his primary-care physician for management. He took no prescription medications. His friend described his memory as "not good", with gradual deterioration in the previous year. He misplaced important papers in his home, including tax forms (although he eventually found and completed them). He forgot appointments, requiring the friend to provide reminders. She no longer was comfortable with his driving; he experienced several "fender-benders" and had been involved in an accident. He continued to read books, but they were less challenging than previously (he no longer participated in the book club owing to hearing loss). He continued to play chess and card games but in a "less organized manner". He continued to do well on the clinical measures (an error in calculation was ascribed to his poor hearing).

Several months prior to his assessment at the age of 88 years, he attempted suicide (cutting his wrists), indicating that he did not want to be "debilitated"; he was hospitalized for treatment of depression. He used a walker because of unsteadiness. He again was hospitalized 3 months prior to assessment for pneumonia; following discharge, he ceased driving and moved to the residence of the collateral source. He was unable to learn the operation of her microwave oven in spite of repeated instructions. Although he still played chess, he relinquished card playing and no longer read books. He needed prompting to change his clothes and was a messier eater. He again weighed 65 kg (143 lbs); he was on a selective serotonin reuptake inhibitor (SSRI) and was not currently depressed. He again did well on the brief clinical cognitive measures except for a single error in calculation. The diagnosis was AD at this and both subsequent assessments. At 89 years of age, he was attending an adult day-care program twice weekly. He continued to live with his friend who supervised his activities; for example, she now assisted him with his household finances (he had double-paid some bills and no longer could balance his checkbook).

His final assessment was at the age of 90 years. He continued to live with his friend. He experienced swallowing difficulty with occasional aspiration. In addition to the SSRI (depression was stable), he was receiving monthly injections of vitamin B12. He now had relinquished all participation in his finances. He frequently was repetitious. On the brief clinical measures, he was disoriented for the date, day of the week, and season and made an error in calculation; however, he still recalled all five items in a memory phrase, drew a clock normally, and serially subtracted 3 from 20.

He entered a nursing home 4 months after this assessment because of difficulty with ambulation and increasing physical needs. A bladder tumor necessitated an indwelling catheter. He would forget visits from his friend shortly afterwards. However, he recited poetry from memory, read the newspaper, and enjoyed discussing current events. Albeit with diminished skills, he played chess until 2 weeks before death. He developed respiratory failure, entered a hospice program, and died at 91 years of age, one year after his last assessment. His clinical course is summarized in the Table 7.2, while Figure 7.2 plots psychometric factor score and CDR against time of testing.

Neuropathological examination revealed the presence of neocortical plaques and neurofibrillary tangles in densities sufficient for a histopathological diagnosis of AD (Figure 7.3).

Comment

This exceptionally high-functioning individual entered the longitudinal study at the age of 69 years as a non-demented control participant. There was no indication of any cognitive problem or complaint until his 9th annual assessment (age 78 years), when he first reported difficulty recalling names. Although he remained capable of meeting the cognitive demands of his many high- level activities and performed

TABLE 7.2 Case report 2: Timeline of clinical milestones

| Assessment | Age (years) | Report of cognitive problem | | Cognitive test performance | | | | | |
		Collateral source	Subject	WMS logical memory (9±2)	Digit span-backwards (5±1)	Mini-mental state exam (28.9±1.3)	Short Blessed test (1.3±2.1)	CDR	Clinical diagnosis
1	69	No problem	No problem	14.5	7	–	–	0	Non-demented
9	78	No problem	Forgetful	11.5	7	–	2	0	Non-demented
12	81	Forgetfulness; errors in tax return	Forgetful					0	Non-demented
15	84	Repetitious; misplacement; reasoning "less clear"	Forgetful	12	6	–	0	0.5	Incipient AD
19	88	Impaired; CS monitors finances	Forgetful; S/P two suicide attempts; lives with CS	9.5	6	29	2	1	AD
20	90	Impaired	Nursing home	7.5	6	27	0	0.5	AD
	91			Expiration summary				1	AD

CDR = clinical dementia rating (0 = no dementia, 0.5 = very mild dementia, 1 = mild dementia); AD = Alzheimer's disease; WMS = Wechsler memory scale; Mean scores of nondemented subjects in the same study as this individual are shown in parentheses for each measure. Higher scores indicate better performance for all measures except the short Blessed test, where lower scores are better.

brief cognitive testing without errors, cognitive complaints persisted at all subsequent assessments. His collateral source did not detect memory problems until years later. Informants rather than affected individuals typically recognize cognitive changes that herald dementia, but rarely may an individual with preserved insight self-detect these changes before they are apparent to anyone else.

Dementia (incipient AD) was not diagnosed until 6 years after his initial complaint. At the time of initial diagnosis, he had no deficits on brief cognitive testing or on psychometric performance, but the collateral source reported the characteristic features of frequent repetition and misplacement of items. Although a gradual decline in psychometric performance occurred from the age of 69 to 84 years, it was very mild, and at the time of dementia diagnosis his performance still was more than one standard deviation better than the mean performance of a non-demented cohort (Table 7.2). It is possible that the slow decline in performance reflected underlying preclinical AD, although other cases of pathologically confirmed preclinical AD have not demonstrated this decline. Alternatively, the very mild decline may simply represent cognitive change associated with normal aging. The precipitous decline in psychometric performance denoting definite impairment did not occur until 4 years after initial clinical recognition of dementia (Figure 7.2).

Dementia is a clinical diagnosis, based on a decline in cognitive abilities sufficient to interfere with the individual's accustomed activities of daily living, and is not determined by neuropsychological "cut-off" scores. The key elements are *change* from prior levels of

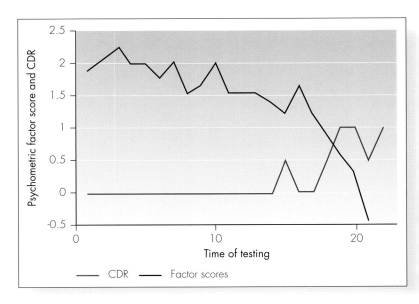

FIGURE 7.2 Case study 2: Longitudinal cognitive performance and dementia severity.

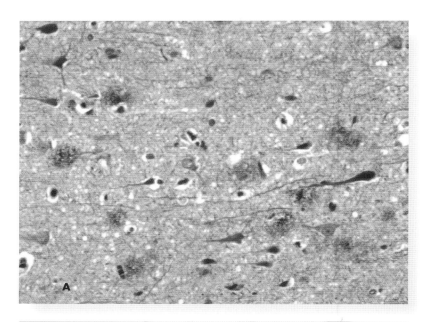

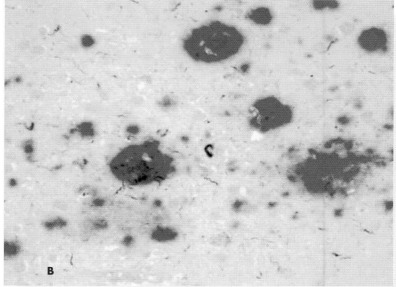

FIGURE 7.3 Case report 2: early-stage AD midfrontal cortex. **(A)** Amyloid plaques and tangles are visualized with the Bielschowsky stain at 400x magnification. **(B)** Dual immunostaining (1005 Ab + PHF-1 tau) reveals amyloid (*red*) and tau (*black*) pathology, 400x magnification.

cognitive function and *impaired everyday performance*. In this subject, the diagnosis was based on the reports of impaired conduct of his everyday activities (e.g. errors in tax return) because of declining cognitive function, even with his continued "normal" performance on cognitive measures. Detection of dementia depends on the quality of the information about the individual's functional performance, particularly any interference caused by cognitive changes, and the diagnostic threshold of the clinician.

Dementia in this individual at the age of 84 years clearly was very mild. Indeed, he did not meet current criteria for MCI because his performance on episodic memory and all other cognitive measures was not impaired. Interpretation of the same reports of very subtle cognitive deficits at the next two annual assessments by different clinicians was that they were in the range of "normal" (CDR 0); even 3 years later, dementia was considered "uncertain" by another clinician. A large "cognitive reserve" may allow functional declines owing to AD to be relatively masked or compensated for several years. However, clinical and functional deterioration eventually occurred in this individual, to the point that his ability to carry out everyday activities clearly was impaired (driving accidents; errors with the checkbook; inability to operate appliances; need for supervision in dressing; and cessation of independent living 3 years before death). The original clinical diagnosis of AD at 84 years of age, at a time when he was insufficiently impaired even to be considered as MCI, was supported both by his subsequent clinical course and by the post-mortem findings.

He experienced depression 2 years after the initial suspicion of AD, possibly because he retained insight into his cognitive deficits and their implications. It is unlikely that depression contributed significantly to his dementia: There was no evidence of depression when dementia first was detected, and dementia continued to progress after depression was stabilized with treatment. Suicide rarely occurs in AD. The suicide attempt in this subject further suggests that his insight was remarkably preserved.

Case report 3: Memory complaints associated with non-demented aging

This woman initially was evaluated at the age of 68 years (June 14, 1985). The subject, a former registered nurse, had a remarkable family history of dementia. Her mother died aged 65 years old with dementia; two of the mother's three sisters and one of her two brothers also were demented. The subject had 12 siblings: 8 sisters and 4 brothers. Of the subject's ten siblings who survived to adulthood, six had dementia of the Alzheimer type. (Alzheimer's disease was confirmed by autopsy in three.) The age at onset (AAO) of dementia in these six siblings ranged from 55 to 86 years; the mean AAO was 73 years. The subject enjoyed excellent health and used no prescription medications. She had sustained head injuries in an automobile accident in 1968, with brief loss of consciousness, and required plastic surgery for facial lacerations; however, she did not have neurological sequela. The initial evaluation disclosed no complaints by the subject or the collateral source (her daughter) of memory or other cognitive impairment. The subject performed brief cognitive tests without any problems. The neurological examination was unremarkable. The CDR was 0.

The CDR scores remained 0 through each of her next five annual assessments. She remained in good physical health. She was very active in her church (serving on several committees), in a senior citizens organization, and in a group of former nursing colleagues.

At her seventh annual assessment at the age of 75 years, the new collateral source was her non-demented sister. The subject had had arthroscopic surgery for right rotator cuff damage 6 months earlier, but still did not require any prescription drugs. The sister reported "barely noticeable" memory problems for the subject for the previous 8 years, including difficulty in remembering dates, occasionally neglecting to turn off her stove burner, and rarely forgetting minor appointments. The collateral source, however, did not believe that these problems interfered with her daily activities. There was no indication of depression. The subject, as before, performed all brief cognitive tests without error. Based on the collateral source's report of "memory problems", the subject was rated as CDR 0.5; dementia was considered "questionable".

The same sister remained the collateral source at the next assessment, when the subject was 76 years old. Again the collateral source reported trivial, inconsistent memory problems that did not interfere with daily activities; the subject's brief cognitive performance remained normal. She was again rated CDR 0.5 with "questionable" dementia; the examiner reported that the questionable impairment "may not progress and may represent normal aging". A very similar history was obtained from the same collateral source at the next assessment, when the subject was 77 years old. The subject remained "extremely active" in card groups and organizations; she cared for a 4-year-old grandchild; she frequently attended movies; and she managed her own finances. Brief cognitive performance was intact. Although the CDR again was CDR 0.5, the examiner noted that the "questionable changes" and "subtle problems reported by the collateral source may represent age-related changes".

Another collateral source (daughter-in-law) came at the next assessment, when the subject was 78 years old. The daughter-in-law reported "no problems" with the subject's memory or thinking. The subject performed brief cognitive tests perfectly. The CDR was 0 (no dementia). She remained CDR 0 at all subsequent assessments through to the age of 84 years. After the age of 78 years, she developed arthritis (treated with a non-steroidal anti-inflammatory drug), hypertension (treated), and Guillain-Barre syndrome with full recovery. She maintained involvement in many activities, including Bible study groups, senior-citizen groups, quilting parties, pinochle, and travel (she drove, including for long trips). She continued to manage her investments and household finances. She performed the brief cognitive tests correctly at all assessments (Table 7.3). Figure 7.4 plots psychometric factor score and CDR against time of testing.

TABLE 7.3 Case report 3: Cognitive test performance

Assessment	Age (years)	WMS logical memory (9±2)	Digit span- back- wards (5±1)	Mini- mental state exam (28.9±1.3)	Short Blessed test (1.3±2.1)	CDR	Clinical diagnosis
1	68	6.5	5	–	2	0	Non-demented
6	74	9.5	6	–	0	0	Non-demented
7	75	7.5	6	–	0	0.5	Questionable dementia
8	76	11.5	7	–	0	0.5	Questionable dementia
9	77	9.0	6	–	2	0.5	Questionable dementia
10	78	8.5	4	–	0	0	Non-demented
12	80	9.0	4	30	0	0	Non-demented
15	83	10.5	5	29	2	0	Non-demented
16	84	7.0	6	30	0	0	Non-demented

CDR = clinical dementia rating (0 = no dementia, 0.5 = very mild dementia, 1 = mild dementia);
AD = Alzheimer's disease; WMS = Wechsler memory scale; Mean scores of nondemented subjects in the same
study as this individual are shown in parentheses for each measure. Higher scores indicate better performance for
all measures except the short Blessed test, where lower scores are better.

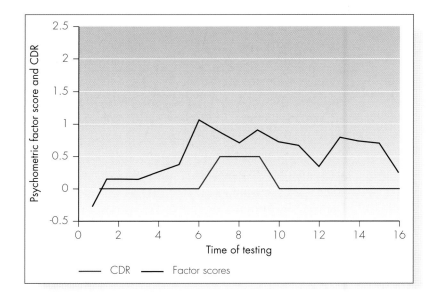

FIGURE 7.4 Case study 3: Longitudinal cognitive performance and dementia severity.

She unexpectedly died in her sleep, 4 months after her last assessment and one week after her 85th birthday. At a Christmas party a few days before her death, she distributed individual gifts (all appropriate) that she had purchased for each of her 7 children, 20 grandchildren, and 14 great-grandchildren.

Neuropathological examination revealed very rare neocortical diffuse plaques (Figure 7.5) and sparse neurofibillary tangles, limited to medial temporal cortex. The lesion densities fell far short of criteria for AD, and the neuropathological diagnosis was "normal brain".

Comment

Clinicians must evaluate the appropriateness of the subjective reports of collateral sources. This subject's initial collateral source (daughter) reported no cognitive difficulty, nor did the third collateral source (daughter-in-law). Combined with the normal performance of the subject on brief cognitive testing at all times, the CDR 0 scores based on these reports appear entirely reasonable. The second collateral source (the subject's sister), however, was concerned about memory "problems". Characteristic features of dementia of the Alzheimer type, such as frequent repetition and misplacement of items, were not reported, nor did the collateral source consider the "problems" sufficient to interfere with the subject's everyday performance. Hence, the subject did not meet criteria for dementia. It also is instructive that the collateral source found the "problems" to be "barely noticeable" and inconsistent. This collateral source may have been hypersensitive to cognitive changes associated with non-demented aging and perhaps over concerned with their importance. Although speculative, the sister may have been overly sensitized by the presence of AD in six of her siblings to any memory lapse of the subject as she approached the average AAO of dementia for their family. This case illustrates that the clinician must weigh carefully any factors that could influence the collateral source to report cognitive impairment, particulary when the report is discrepant with sustained normal cognitive and functional performance of the subject (Table 7.3).

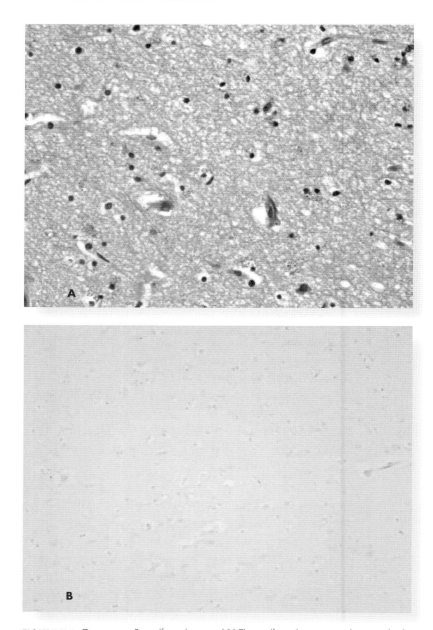

FIGURE 7.5 Case report 3: midfrontal cortex. **(A)** The midfrontal cortex is without amyloid plaques and tangles; Bielschowsky stain at 400x magnification. **(B)** Amyloid and tau pathology are absent with dual immunostaining (1005 Aβ + PHF-1 tau); 400x magnification.

References

1. Ganguli M, Dodge HH, Shen C, DeKosky ST. Mild cognitive impairment, amnestic type: An epidemiologic study. Neurology. 2004;63(1):115–121.

2. Boyle PA, Wilson RS, Aggarwal NT, Tang Y, Bennett DA. Mild cognitive impairment: Risk of Alzheimer disease and rate of cognitive decline. Neurology. August 8, 2006 2006;67(3):441–445.

3. Markesbery WR, Schmitt FA, Kryscio RJ, Davis DG, Smith CD, Wekstein DR. Neuropathologic substrate of mild cognitive impairment.[see comment]. Archives of Neurology. Jan 2006;63(1): 38–46.

4. Bennett DA, Schneider JA, Bienias JL, Evans DA, Wilson RS. Mild cognitive impairment is related to Alzheimer disease pathology and cerebral infarctions. Neurology. March 8, 2005 2005;64(5):834–841.

5. Petersen RC, Parisi JE, Dickson DW, et al. Neuropathologic Features of Amnestic Mild Cognitive Impairment. Arch Neurol. May 1, 2006 2006;63(5):665–672.

6. Jicha GA, Parisi JE, Dickson DW, et al. Neuropathologic Outcome of Mild Cognitive Impairment Following Progression to Clinical Dementia. Arch Neurol. May 1, 2006 2006;63(5):674–681.

7. Barnes DE, Alexopoulos GS, Lopez OL, Williamson JD, Yaffe K. Depressive symptoms, vascular disease, and mild cognitive impairment: findings from the Cardiovascular Health Study. Archives of General Psychiatry. Mar 2006;63(3):273–279.

8. Geda YE, Knopman DS, Mrazek DA, et al. Depression, apolipoprotein E genotype, and the incidence of mild cognitive impairment: a prospective cohort study. Archives of Neurology. Mar 2006;63(3): 435–440.

9. Verghese J, LeValley A, Derby C, et al. Leisure activities and the risk of amnestic mild cognitive impairment in the elderly.[see comment]. Neurology. Mar 28 2006;66(6):821–827.

10. Mintun MA, LaRossa GN, Sheline YI, et al. [11C]PIB in a non-demented population: Potential antecedent marker of Alzheimer disease. Neurology. August 8, 2006 2006;67(3):446–452.

11. Petersen RC, Thomas RG, Grundman M, et al. Vitamin E and donepezil for the treatment of mild cognitive impairment. [see comment]. New England Journal of Medicine. Jun 9 2005;352(23): 2379-2388.

12. Flicker C, Ferris SH, Reisberg B. Mild cognitive impairment in the elderly: Predictors of dementia. Neurology 1991; 41:1006–1009.

13. Graham JE, Rockwood K, Beattie BL et al. Prevalence and severity of cognitive impairment with and without dementia in an elderly population. J Lancet 1997; 349:1793–1796.

14. Di Carlo A, Baldereschi M, Amaducci L et al. Cognitive impairment without dementia in older people: Prevalence, vascular risk factors, impact on disability. The Italian longitudinal study on aging. J Am Geriatr Soc 2000; 48:775–782.

15. Kral VA. Senescent forgetfulness: Benign and malignant. Can Med Assoc J 1962; 86:257–260.

16. Crook TH, Bartus RT. Age-associated memory impairment: Proposed diagnostic criteria and measures of clinical change – Report of a National Institute of Mental Health work group. Dev Neuropsychol 1986; 2:261–276.

17. Levy R. Aging-associated cognitive decline. Int Psychogeriatr 1994; 6:63–68.

18. Bennett DA, Wilson RS, Schneider JA et al. Natural history of mild cognitive impairment in older persons. Neurology. 2002; 59:198

19. Ritchie K., Touchon J. Mild cognitive impairment: conceptual basis and current nosological status. J Lancet 2000; 355:225–228.

20. Petersen RC, Smith GE, Waring SC et al. Mild cognitive impairment – Clinical characterization and outcome. Arch Neurol 1999; 56:303–308.

21. Golomb J, Kluger A, Ferris SH. Mild cognitive impairment: Identifying and treating the earliest stages of Alzheimer's disease. Neurosci News 2000; 3:46–53.

22. Petersen RC. Normal aging, mild cognitive impairment, and early Alzheimer's disease. Neurologist 1995; 1:326–344.

23. Larrieu S, Letenneur L, Orgogozo JM et al. Incidence and outcome of mild cognitive impairment in a population-based prospective cohort. Neurology 2002; 59:1594–1599.

24. Ritchie K, Artero S, Touchon J. Classification criteria for mild cognitive impairment. A population-based validation study. Neurology 2001; 56:37–42.

25. Unverzagt FW, Gao S, Baiyewu O et al. Prevalence of cognitive impairment: Data from the Indianapolis Study of Health and Aging. Neurology 2001; 57:1655–1662.

26. Lopez OL, Jagust WJ, Dulberg C et al. Risk Factors for Mild Cognitive Impairment in the Cardiovascular Health Study Cognition Study: Part 2. Arch Neurol 2003; 60:1394–1399.

27. Ebly EM, Hogan DB, Parhad IM. Cognitive impairment in the non-demented elderly. Results from the Canadian Study of Health and Aging. Arch Neurol 1995; 52:612–619.

28. Luis CA, Loewenstein DA, Acevedo A, Barker WW, Duara R. Mild cognitive impairment: Directions for future research. Neurology 2003; 61:438–444.

29. Bowen J, Teri L, Kukull W et al. Progression to dementia in patients with isolated memory loss. J Lancet. 1997; 349:763-765

30. Dawe B, Procter A, Philpot M. Concepts of mild memory impairment in the elderly and their relationship to dementia: A review. Int J Geriatr Psychiatry 1992; 7:473–479.

31. Tierney MC, Snow WG, Reid DW, Zorzitto ML, Fisher RH. Psychometric differentiation of dementia. Replication and extension of the findings of Storandt and coworkers. Arch Neurol 1987; 44:720–722.

32. Carr DB, Gray S, Baty J, Morris JC. The value of informant vs. individual's complaints of memory impairment in early dementia. Neurology 2000; 55:1724–1726.

33. Koss E, Patterson MB, Ownby R, Stuckey JC, Whitehouse PJ. Memory evaluation in Alzheimer's disease: Caregivers' appraisals and objective testing. Arch Neurol 1993; 50:92–97.

34. McGlone J, Gupta S, Humphrey D et al. Screening for early dementia using memory complaints from patients and relatives. Arch Neurol 1990; 47:1189–1193.

35. Jorm AF. Methods of screening for dementia: A meta-analysis of studies comparing an informant questionnaire with a brief cognitive test. Alzheimer Dis Assoc Disord 1997; 11:158–162.

36. Tierney MC, Szalai JP, Snow WG, Fisher RH. The prediction of Alzheimer disease. Arch Neurol 1996; 53:423–427.

37. Grundman M, Petersen RC, Ferris SH et al. Mild cognitive impairment can be distinguished from Alzheimer disease and normal aging for clinical trials. Arch Neurol 2004; 61:59–66.

38. Evans DA, Funkenstein HH, Albert MS et al. Prevalence of Alzheimer's disease in a community population of older persons: Higher than previously reported. JAMA 1989; 262:2551–2556.

39. Devanand DP, Folz M, Gorlyn M, Moeller JR, Stern Y. Questionable dementia: Clinical course and predictors of outcome. J Am Geriatr Soc 1997; 45:321–328.

40. Galasko D, Klauber MR, Hofstetter R. The mini-mental state examination in the early diagnosis of Alzheimer's disease. Arch Neurol 1990; 47:49–52.

41. Herlitz A, Small BJ, Fratiglioni L et al. Detection of mild dementia in community surveys. Arch Neurol 1997; 54:319–324.

42. Morris JC, McKeel DW, Jr., Storandt M et al. Very mild Alzheimer's disease: Informant-based clinical, psychometric, and pathologic distinction from normal aging. Neurology 1991; 41:469–478.

43. Ebly EM, Parhad IM, Hogan DB, Fung TS. Prevalence and types of dementia in the very old – Results from the Canadian Study of Health and Aging. Neurology 1994; 44:1593–1600.

44. Craik FIM. Memory functions in normal aging. In: Yanagihara T, Petersen RC, editors. Memory Disorders, Research and Clinical Practice. New York: Marcel Dekker, 1991: 347–367.

45. Salthouse TA. The aging of working memory. Neuropsychology 1994; 8:535–543.

46. Schaie KW. The hazards of cognitive aging. Gerontologist 1989; 29:484–493.

47. Salthouse TA. What do adult age differences in the digit symbol substitution test reflect? J Gerontol 1992; 47:P121–P128.

48. Rubin EH, Storandt M, Miller JP et al. Influence of age on clinical and psychometric assessment of subjects with very mild or mild dementia of the Alzheimer type. Arch Neurol 1993; 50:380–383.

49. Sliwinski M, Lipton RB, Buschke H, Stewart W. The effects of preclinical dementia on estimates of normal cognitive functioning in aging. J Gerontol 1996; 51B:P217–P225.

50. Howieson DB, Dame A, Camicioli R et al. Cognitive markers preceding Alzheimer's dementia in the healthy oldest old. J Am Geriatr Soc 1997; 45:584–589.

51. Rubin EH, Storandt M, Miller JP et al. A prospective study of cognitive function and onset of dementia in cognitively healthy elders. Arch Neurol 1998; 55:395–401.

52. Storandt M, Grant EA, Miller JP, Morris JC. Rates of progression in mild cognitive impairment and early Alzheimer's disease. Neurology 2002; 59:1034–1041.

53. Morris JC, Edland S, Clark C et al. The Consortium to Establish a Registry for Alzheimer's Disease (CERAD). Part IV. Rates of cognitive change in the longitudinal assessment of probable Alzheimer's disease. Neurology 1993; 43:2457–2465.

54. Crystal H, Dickson D, Fuld P et al. Clinico-pathologic studies in dementia: Nondemented subjects with pathologically confirmed Alzheimer's disease. Neurology 1988; 38:1682–1687.

55. Haan MN, Shemanki L, Jagust WJ, Manolio TA. The role of APOE ε4 in modulating effects of other risk factors for cognitive decline in elderly persons. JAMA 1999; 282:40–46.

56. Berg L, McKeel DW, Jr., Miller JP et al. Clinicopathologic studies in cognitively healthy aging and Alzheimer disease: Relation of histologic markers to dementia severity, age, sex, and apolipoprotein E genotype. Arch Neurol 1998; 55:326–335.

57. Gomez-Isla T, Price JL, Morris JC, Growdon JH. Profound loss of layer II entorhinal cortex neurons occurs in very mild Alzheimer's disease. J Neurosci 1996; 16:4491–4500.

58. Price JL, Morris JC. Tangles and plaques in nondemented aging and "preclinical" Alzheimer's disease. Ann Neurol 1999; 45:358–368.

59. Mirra SS, Heyman A, McKeel DW et al. The Consortium to Establish a Registry for Alzheimer's Disease (CERAD). Part II. Standardization of the neuropathologic assessment of Alzheimer's disease. Neurology 1991; 41:479–486.

60. Khachaturian ZS. Diagnosis of Alzheimer's disease. Arch Neurol 1985; 42:1097–1105.

61. National Institute on Aging, Reagan Institute Working Group on Diagnostic Criteria for the Neuropathological Assessment of Alzheimer's Disease. Consensus recommendations for the post-mortem diagnosis of Alzheimer's disease. Neurobiol Aging 1997; 18:S1–S2.

62. Gellerstedt N. Zur Kenntnis der Hirneveränderungen bei der normalen Altersinvolution. Ups LaKaref Forh 1933; 38:193.

63. Tomlinson BE, Blessed G, Roth M. Observations on the brains of non-demented old people. J Neurol Sci 1968; 7:331–356.

64. Tomlinson BE, Blessed G, Roth M. Observations on the brains of demented old people. J Neurol Sci 1970; 11:205–242.

65. Blessed G, Tomlinson BE, Roth M. The association between quantitative measures of dementia and of senile change in the cerebral grey matter of the elderly subjects. Br J Psychiatry 1968; 114:797–811.

66. Arriagada PV, Marzloff K, Hyman BT. Distribution of Alzheimer-type pathologic changes in nondemented elderly individuals matches the pattern in Alzheimer's disease. Neurology 1992; 42:1681–1688.

67. Braak H, Braak E. Frequency of stages of Alzheimer-related lesions in different age categories. Neurobiol Aging 1997; 18:351–357.

68. Haroutunian V, Purohit DP, Perl DP et al. Neurofibrillary tangles in nondemented elderly subjects and mild Alzheimer disease. Arch Neurol 1999; 56:713–718.

69. Morris JC, Storandt M, McKeel DW et al. Cerebral amyloid deposition and diffuse plaques in "normal" aging: Evidence for presymptomatic and very mild Alzheimer's disease. Neurology 1996; 46:707–719.

70. Troncoso JC, Martin LJ, Dal Forno G, Kawas CH. Neuropathology in controls and demented subjects from the Baltimore Longitudinal Study of Aging. Neurobiol Aging 1996; 17:365–371.

71. Haroutunian V, Perl DP, Purohit DP et al. Regional distribution of neuritic plaques in the nondemented elderly and subjects with very mild Alzheimer disease. Arch Neurol 1998; 55:1185–1191.

72. Morris JC, Storandt M, Miller JP et al. Mild cognitive impairment represents early-stage Alzheimer's disease. Arch Neurol 2001; 58:397–405.

73. DeKosky ST, Ikonomovic MD, Styren SD et al. Upregulation of choline acetyltransferase activity in hippocampus and frontal cortex of elderly subjects with mild cognitive impairment. Ann Neurol 2002; 51:145–155.

74. Kordower JH, Chu Y, Stebbins GT et al. Loss and atrophy of layer II entorhinal cortex neurons in elderly people with mild cognitive impairment. Ann Neurol 2001; 49:202–213.

75. Tierney MC, Szalai JP, Snow WG et al. Prediction of probable Alzheimer's disease in memory-impaired patients: A prospective longitudinal study. Neurology. 1996; 46:661-665

76. Dik MG, Jonker C, Bouter LM et al. APOE-ε is associated with memory decline in cognitively impaired elderly. Neurology 2000; 54:1492–1497.

77. Lyketsos CG, Lopez O, Jones B et al. Prevalence of neuropsychiatric symptoms in dementia and mild cognitive impairment: Results from the cardiovascular health study. JAMA 2002; 288:1475–1483.

78. Jack CR, Petersen RC, Xu YE et al. Medial temporal atrophy on MRI in normal aging and very mild Alzheimer's disease. Neurology 1997; 49:786–794.

79. Jack CR, Petersen RC, Xu YC et al. Prediction of AD with MRI-based hippocampal volume in mild cognitive impairment. Neurology 1999; 52:1397–1403.

80. Fox NC, Warrington EK, Seiffer AL, Agnew SK, Rossor MN. Presymptomatic cognitive deficits in individuals at risk of familial Alzheimer's disease – A longitudinal prospective study. Brain 1998; 121:1631–1639.

81. Petersen RC, Doody R, Kurz A et al. Current concepts in mild cognitive impairment. Arch Neurol 2001; 58:1985–1992.

82. Laakso MP, Soininen H, Partanen K et al. Volumes of hippocampus, amygdala and frontal lobes in the MRI-based diagnosis of early Alzheimers disease – Correlation with memory functions. J Neural Transm Park Dis Dement Sect 1995; 9:73–86.

83. Murphy DGM, Decarli CD, Daly E et al. Volumetric magnetic-resonance-imaging in men with dementia of the Alzheimer-type – correlations with disease severity. Biol Psychiatry 1993; 34:612–621.

84. Killiany RJ, Moss MB, Sandor T, Tieman J. Temporal lobe regions on magnetic resonance imaging identify patients with early Alzheimer's disease. Arch Neurol 1993; 50:949–954.

85. Du AT, Schuff N, Amend D et al. Magnetic resonance imaging of the entorhinal cortex and hippocampus in mild cognitive impairment and Alzheimer's disease. J Neurol Neurosurg Psychiatry 2001; 71:441–447.

86. Jack CR, Jr., Dickson DW, Parisi JE et al. Antemortem MRI findings correlate with hippocampal neuropathology in typical aging and dementia. Neurology 2002; 58:750–757.

87. Gosche KM, Mortimer JA, Smith CD, Markesbery WR, Snowdon DA. Hippocampal volume as an index of Alzheimer neuropathology: Findings from the Nun Study. Neurology 2002; 58:1476–1482.

88. Silbert LC, Quinn JF, Moore MM et al. Changes in premorbid brain volume predict Alzheimer's disease pathology. Neurology 2003; 61:487–492.

89. Csernansky JG, Wang L, Joshi S et al. Early DAT is distinguished from aging by high dimensional mapping of the hippocampus. Neurology 2000; 55:1636–1643.

90. de Leon MJ, Convit A, Wolf OT et al. Prediction of cognitive decline in normal elderly subjects with 2-[^{18}F]fluoro-2-deoxy-D-glucose/positron-emission tomography (FDG/PET). Proc Natl Acad Sci USA 2001; 98:10966–10971.

91. Silverman DHS, Small GW, Chang CY et al. Positron emission tomography in evaluation of dementia: Regional brain metabolism and long-term outcome. JAMA 2001; 286:2120–2127.

92. Celsis P, Agniel A, Cardebat D et al. Age related cognitive decline: A clinical entity? A longitudinal study of cerebral blood flow and memory performance. J Neurol Neurosurg Psychiatry 1997; 62:601–608.

93. Johnson KA, Jones K, Holman BL et al. Preclinical prediction of Alzheimer's disease using SPECT. Neurology 1998; 50:1563–1571.

94. Anonymous. Consensus conference: Differential diagnosis of dementing diseases. JAMA 1987; 258:3411–3416.

95. Hebert LE, Beckett LA, Scherr PA, Evans DA. Annual incidence of Alzheimer disease in the United States projected to the years 2000 through 2050. Alzheimer Dis Assoc Disord 2001; 15:169–173.

96. Barrett JJ, Haley WE, Harrell LE, Powers RE. Knowledge about Alzheimer disease among primary care physicians, psychologists, nurses, and social workers. Alzheimer Dis Assoc Disord 1997; 11:99–106.

97. Richter RW, Richter BZ. Alzheimer's Disease. London: Mosby, 2002.

98. Knopman DS, DeKosky ST, Cummings JL et al. Practice parameter: Diagnosis of dementia (an evidence-based review). Report of the Quality Standards Subcommittee of the American Academy of Neurology. Neurology 2001; 56:1143–1153.

99. McKhann G, Drachman D, Folstein M et al. Clinical diagnosis of Alzheimer's disease: Report of the NINCDS–ADRDA Work Group under the auspices of Department of Health and Human Services Task Force on Alzheimer's disease. Neurology 1984; 34:939–944.

100. Powlishta K, Storandt M, Hogan E, Grant EA, Morris JC. The effect of depression on psychometric test performance in individuals in the early stages of Alzheimer's disease. Arch Neurol 2004 (In press).

101. Bolla KI, Lindgren KN, Bonaccorsy C, Bleecker ML. Memory complaints in older adults: Fact or fiction? Arch Neurol 1991; 48:61–64.

102. Flicker C, Ferris SH, Reisberg B. A longitudinal study of cognitive function in elderly persons with subjective memory complaints. J Am Geriatr Soc 1993; 41:1029–1032.

103. Snowdon DA, Greiner LH, Mortimer JA et al. Brain infarction and the clinical expression of Alzheimer disease. JAMA 1997; 277:813–817.

104. Chui H, Zhang Q. Evaluation of dementia: A systematic study of the usefulness of the American Academy of Neurology's practice parameters. Neurology 1997; 49:925–935.

105. McMahon PM, Araki SS, Neumann PJ, Harris GJ, Gazelle GS. Cost-effectiveness of functional imaging tests in the diagnosis of Alzheimer disease. Radiology 2000; 217:58–68.

106. Forsell Y, Winblad B. Major depression in a population of demented and nondemented older people: Prevalence and correlates. J Am Geriatr Soc 1998; 46:27–30.

107. Clarfield AM. The reversible dementias: Do they reverse? Ann Intern Med 1988; 109:476–486.

108. American Academy of Neurology/Quality Standards Subcommittee. Practice parameter for diagnosis and evaluation of dementia. Neurology 1994; 44:2203–2206.

109. Folstein MF, Folstein SE, McHugh PR. Mini-mental state: A practical method for grading the cognitive state of patients for the clinicians. J Psychiatr Res 1975; 12:189–198.

110. Doraiswamy PM, Krishen A, Stallone F et al. Cognitive performance on the Alzheimer's disease assessment scale: Effect of education. Neurology 1995; 45:1980–1984.

111. Manly JJ, Jacobs DM, Sano M et al. Cognitive test performance among nondemented elderly African Americans and whites. Neurology 1998; 50:1238–1245.

112. Petersen RC, Stevens JC, Ganguli M et al. Practice parameter: Early detection of dementia: Mild cognitive impairment (an evidence-based review) Report of the Quality Standards Subcommittee of the American Academy of Neurology. Neurology 2001; 56:1133–1142.

113. Ganguli M, Belle S, Ratcliff G et al. Sensitivity and specificity for dementia of population-based criteria for cognitive impairment: the MoVIES project. J Gerontol 1993; 48:M152–M161.

114. Kukull WA, Larson EB, Teri L et al. The mini-mental state examination score and the clinical diagnosis of dementia. J Clin Epidemiol 1994; 47:1061–1067.

115. Agrell B, Dehlin O. The clock-drawing test. Age Ageing 1998; 27:399–403.

116. Shulman K. Clock-drawing: Is it the ideal cognitive screening test? Int J Geriatr Psychiatry 2000; 15:548–561.

117. Powlishta KK, Von Dras DD, Stanford A et al. The clock drawing test is a poor screen for very mild dementia. Neurology 2002; 59:898–903.

118. Solomon PR, Hirschoff A, Kelly B et al. A 7 minute neurocognitive screening battery highly sensitive to Alzheimer's disease. Arch Neurol 1998; 55:349–355.

119. Morris JC. The Clinical Dementia Rating (CDR): Current version and scoring rules. Neurology 1993; 43:2412–2414.

120. Hughes CP, Berg L, Danziger WL, Coben LA, Martin RL. A new clinical scale for the staging of dementia. Br J Psychiatry 1982; 140:566–572.

121. Burke WJ, Miller JP, Rubin EH et al. Reliability of the Washington University Clinical Dementia Rating. Arch Neurol 1988; 45:31–32.

122. McCulla MM, Coats M, Van Fleet N et al. Reliability of clinical nurse specialists in the staging of dementia. Arch Neurol 1989; 46:1210–1211.

123. Morris JC, McKeel DW, Fulling K, Torack RM, Berg L. Validation of clinical diagnostic criteria for Alzheimer's disease. Ann Neurol 1988; 24:17–22.

124. Reisberg B, Ferris SH, deLeon MJ. The Global deterioration scale for assessment of primary degenerative dementia. Am J Psychiatry 1982; 139:1136–1139.

125. O'Connor DW, Pollitt PA, Roth M, Brook PB, Reiss BB. Memory complaints and impairment in normal, depressed, and demented elderly persons identified in a community survey. Arch Gen Psychiatry 1990; 47:224–227.

126. Burt DB, Zembar MJ, Niederehe G. Depression and memory impairment: a meta-analysis of the association, its pattern, and specificity. Psychol Bull 1995; 117:285–305.

127. Forsell Y, Jorm AF, Winblad B. Association of age, sex, cognitive dysfunction, and disability with major depressive symptoms in an elderly sample. Am J Psychiatry 1994; 151:1600–1604.

128. Rabbitt P, Donlan C, Watson P, McInnes L, Bent N. Unique and interactive effects of depression, age, socioeconomic advantage, and gender on cognitive performance of normal healthy older people. Psychol Aging 1995; 10:307–313.

129. Reifler BV. Pre-dementia. J Am Geriatr Soc 1997; 45:776–777.

130. Reifler BV. A case of mistaken identity: Pseudodementia is really predementia. J Am Geriatr Soc 2000; 48:593–594.

131. Devanand DP, Miller L, Richards M et al. The Columbia University scale for psychopathology in Alzheimer's disease. Arch Neurol 1992; 49:371–376.

132. Wragg RE, Jeste DV. Overview of depression and psychosis in Alzheimer's disease. Am J Psychiatry 1989; 146:577–587.

133. Kral VA. The relationship between senile dementia (Alzheimer type) and depression. Can J Psychiatry 1983; 28:304–306.

134. Wilson RS, Barnes LL, de Leon CM et al. Depressive symptoms and risk of Alzheimer's disease in older persons. Ann Neurol 2001; 50:S45.

135. Zubenko GS, Moossy J. Major depression in primary dementia: Clinical and neuropathologic correlates. Arch Neurol 1988; 45:1182–1186.

136. Ritchie K, Touchon J, Ledesert B. Progressive disability in senile dementia is accelerated in the presence of depression. Int J Geriatr Psychiatry 1998; 13:459–461.

137. McNeil JK. Neuropsychological characteristics of the dementia syndrome of depression: onset, resolution, and three-year follow-up. Clin Neuropsychol 1999; 13:136–146.

138. Nagy Z, Esiri MM, Jobst KA, et al. The effects of additional pathology on the cognitive deficit in Alzheimer disease. J Neuropathol Exp Neurol 1997; 56:165–170.

139. Trojanowski JQ, Lee VMY. Aggregation of neurofilament and α-synuclein proteins in Lewy bodies. Arch Neurol 1998; 55:151–152.

140. McKeith IG, Galasko D, Kosaka K et al. Consensus guidelines for the clinical and pathologic diagnosis of dementia with Lewy bodies (DLB): Report of the consortium on DLB international workshop. Neurology 1996; 47:1113–1124.

141. Marder K, Tang M-X, Cote L, Stern Y, Mayeux R. The frequency and associated risk factors for dementia in patients with Parkinson's disease. Arch Neurol 1995; 52:695–701.

142. Small GW, Rabins PV, Barry PP et al. Diagnosis and treatment of Alzheimer disease and related disorders: Consensus statement of the American Association for Geriatric Psychiatry, the Alzheimer's Association, and the American Geriatrics Society. JAMA 1997; 278:1363–1371.

143. del Ser T, Bermejo F, Portera A et al. Vascular dementia: A clinicopathological study. J Neurol Sci 1990; 96:1–17.

144. Nolan KA, Lino MM, Seligmann AW, Blass JP. Absence of vascular dementia in an autopsy series from a dementia clinic. J Am Geriatr Soc 1998; 46:597–604.

145. Hulette C, Nochlin D, McKeel DW et al. Clinical-neuropathologic findings in multi-infarct dementia: A report of six autopsied cases. Neurology 1997; 48:668–672.

146. Rosen WG, Terry RD, Fuld PA, Katzman R, Peck A. Pathological verification of ischemic score in differentiation of dementias. Ann Neurol 1980; 7:486–488.

147. Neary D, Snowden JS, Gustafson L et al. Frontotemporal lobar degeneration: A consensus on clinical diagnostic criteria. Neurology 1998; 51:1546–1554.

148. Mann DMA. Dementia of frontal type and dementias with subcortical gliosis. Brain Pathol 1998; 8:325–338.

149. Ratnavalli E, Brayne C, Dawson K, Hodges JR. The prevalence of frontotemporal dementia. Neurology 2002; 58:1615–1621.

150. Dickson DW. Neurodegenerative diseases with cytoskeletal pathology: A biochemical classification. Ann Neurol 1997; 42:541–544.

151. Van Swieten JC, Stevens M, Rosso SM et al. Phenotypic variation in hereditary frontotemporal dementia with tau mutations. Ann Neurol 1999; 46:617–626.

152. Kertesz A, Munoz D. Pick's disease, frontotemporal dementia and pick complex. Arch Neurol 1998; 55:302–304.

153. Touchon J, Ritchie K. Prodromal cognitive disorder in Alzheimer's disease. Int J Geriatr Psychiatry 1999; 14:556–563.

154. Raskind MA, Peskind ER, Wessel T, Yuan W, and the Galantamine USA-1 Study Group. Galantamine in AD: A 6-month randomized, placebo-controlled trial with a 6-month extension. Neurology 2000; 54:2261–2268.

155. Farlow M, Anand R, Messina J, Hartman R, Veach J. A 52-week study of the efficacy of rivastigmine in patients with mild to moderately severe Alzheimer's disease. Eur Neurol 2000; 44:236–241.

156. Scarmeas N, Levy G, Tang MX, Manly J, Stern Y. Influence of leisure activity on the incidence of Alzheimer's Disease. Neurology 2001; 57:2236–2242.

157. Laurin D, Verreault R, Lindsay J, MacPherson K, Rockwood K. Physical activity and risk of cognitive impairment and dementia in elderly persons. Arch Neurol 2001; 58:498–504.

158. Bartus RT, Dean RI, Beer B, Lippa AS. The cholinergic hypothesis of geriatric memory dysfunction. Science 1982; 217:408–414.

159. Davis KL, Mohs RC, Marin D et al. Cholinergic markers in elderly patients with early signs of Alzheimer disease. JAMA 2000; 281:1401–1406.

160. Tiraboschi P, Hansen LA, Alford M et al. The decline in synapses and cholinergic activity is asynchronous in Alzheimer's disease. Neurology 2000; 55:1278–1283.

161. Grutzendler J, Morris JC. Cholinesterase inhibitors for Alzheimer's disease. Drugs 2001; 61:41–52.

162. Farlow M, Gracon SI, Hershey LA et al. A controlled trial of tacrine in Alzheimer's disease. JAMA 1992; 268:2523–2529.

163. Davis KL, Thal LJ, Gamzu ER et al. A double-blind, placebo-controlled multicenter study of tacrine for Alzheimer's disease. N Engl J Med 1992; 327:1253–1259.

164. Knapp MJ, Knopman DS, Solomon PR et al. A 30-week randomized controlled trial of high-dose tacrine in patients with Alzheimer's disease. JAMA 1994; 271:985–991.

165. Thal LJ, Schwartz G, Sano M et al. A multicenter double-blind study of controlled-release physostigmine for the treatment of symptoms secondary to Alzheimer's disease. Neurology 1996; 47:1389–1395.

166. Corey-Bloom J, Anand R, Veach J, for the ENA 713 B352 Study Group. A randomized trial evaluating the efficacy and safety of ENA 713 (rivastigmine tartrate), a new acetylcholinesterase inhibitor, in

patients with mild to moderately severe Alzheimer's disease. Int J Geriatr Psychopharmacol 1998; 1:55–65.

167. Morris JC, Cyrus PA, Orazem J et al. Metrifonate benefits cognitive, behavioral, and global function in patients with Alzheimer's disease. Neurology 1998; 50:1222–1230.

168. Imbimbo BP, Martelli P, Troetel WM et al. Efficacy and safety of eptastigmine for the treatment of patients with Alzheimer's disease. Neurology 1999; 52:700–708.

169. Rosler M, Anand R, Cicin-Sain A et al. Efficacy and safety of rivastigmine in patients with Alzheimer's disease: international randomized controlled trial. BMJ 1999; 318:633–638.

170. Winblad B, Engedal K, Soininen H et al. A 1-year, randomized, placebo-controlled study of donepezil in patients with mild to moderate AD. Neurology 2001; 57:489–495.

171. Mohs RC, Doody RS, Morris JC et al. A 1-year, placebo-controlled preservation of function survival study of donepezil in AD patients. Neurology 2001; 57:481–488.

172. Mohs RC, Doody RS, Morris JC, Ieni JR, Rogers SL, Perdomo CA et al. The preservation of function in Alzheimer's disease: results from a 1-year placebo-controlled study with donepezil. In: Vellas B, Feldman H, Fitten LJ, Winblad B, Giacobini E (eds). Research and Practice in Alzheimer Disease and Cognitive Decline. Paris: Serdi, 2002.

173. Getsios D, Caro JJ, Caro G, Ishak K. Assessment of health economics in Alzheimer's disease (AHEAD). Neurology 2001; 57:972–978.

174. Doody RS, Stevens JC, Beck C et al. Practice parameter: Management of dementia (an evidence-based review) Report of the quality standards subcommittee of the American Academy of Neurology. Neurology 2001; 56:1154–1166.

175. Lipton SA, Rosenberg PA. Excitatory amino acids as a final common pathway for neurologic disorders. N Engl J Med 1994;613–622.

176. Farber NB, Newcomer JW, Olney JW. The glutamate synapse in neuropsychiatric disorders: Focus on schizophrenia and Alzheimer's disease. Prog Brain Res 1998; 116:421–437.

177. Klegeris A, McGeer PL. Beta-amyloid protein enhances macrophage production of oxygen free radicals and glutamate. J Neurosci Res 1997; 49:229–235.

178. Reisberg B, Doody R, Stoffler A et al. Memantine in moderate-to-severe Alzheimer's disease. N Engl J Med 2003; 348:1333–1341.

179. Tariot PN, Farlow MR, Grossberg GT et al. Memantine treatment in patients with moderate to severe Alzheimer disease already

receiving donepezil: A randomized controlled trial. JAMA 2004; 291:317–324.

180. Sano M, Ernesto C, Thomas RG et al. A controlled trial of selegiline, alpha-tocopherol, or both as treatment for Alzheimer's disease. N Engl J Med 1997; 336:1216–1222.

181. Zandi PP, Anthony JC, Khachaturian AS et al. Reduced risk of Alzheimer disease in users of antioxidant vitamin supplements: The Cache County Study. Arch Neurol 2004; 61:82–88.

182. Yaffe K. Hormone therapy and the brain: Deja vu all over again? JAMA 2003; 289:2717–2719.

183. Tang M, Jacobs D, Stern Y. Effect of estrogen during menopause on risk and age at onset of Alzheimer's disease. J Lancet 1996; 348:429–432.

184. Kawas C, Resnick S, Morrison A et al. A prospective study of estrogen replacement therapy and the risk of developing Alzheimer's disease: The Baltimore Longitudinal Study of Aging. Neurology 1997; 48:1517–1521.

185. Zandi PP, Carlson M, Plassman BL et al. Hormone replacement therapy and incidence of Alzheimer disease in older women; The Cache County Study. JAMA 2002; 288:2123–2129.

186. Yaffe K, Sawaya G, Lieberburg I, Grady D. Estrogen therapy in postmenopausal women. JAMA 1998; 279:688–695.

187. Shumaker SA, Legault C, Rapp SR et al. Estrogen plus progestin and the incidence of dementia and mild cognitive impairment in postmenopausal women. The Women's Health Initiative Memory Study: A randomized controlled trial. JAMA 2003; 289:2651–2662.

188. Rapp SR, Espeland MA, Shumaker SA et al. Effect of estrogen plus progestin on global cognitive function in postmenopausal women. JAMA 2003; 289:2663–2672.

189. Wassertheil-Smoller S, Hendrix S, Limacher M et al. Effect of estrogen plus progestin on stroke in postmenopausal women: The Women's Health Initiative: A randomized trial. JAMA 2003; 289:2673–2684.

190. Writing Group for the Women's Health Initiative Investigators. Risks and benefits of estrogen plus progestin in healthy postmenopausal women. JAMA 2002; 288:321–333.

191. Aisen PS, Davis KL. Inflammatory mechanisms in Alzheimer's disease: Implications for therapy. Am J Psychiatry 1994; 151:1105–1113.

192. Singh VK, Guthikonda P. Circulating cytokines in Alzheimer's disease. J Psychiatr Res 1997; 31:657–660.

193. Weaver JD, Huang MH, Albert M. et al. Interleukin-6 and risk of cognitive decline. Neurology 2002; 59:371–378

194. Weggen S, Eriksen JL, Das P et al. A subset of NSAIDs lower amyloidogenic Aβ_{42} independently of cyclooxygenase activity. Nature 2001; 414:212–216.

195. in 't Veld BA, Ruitenberg A, Hofman A et al. Nonsteroidal antiinflammatory drugs and the risk of Alzheimer's disease. N Engl J Med 2001; 345:1515–1521.

196. Aisen PS, Davis KL, Berg MS et al. A randomized controlled trial of prednisone in Alzheimer's disease. Neurology 2000; 54:588–593.

197. Jick H, Zornberg GL, Jick SS, Seshadri S, Drachman DA. Statins and the risk of dementia. J Lancet 2000; 356:1627–1631.

198. Wolozin B, Kellman W, Ruosseau P, Celesia GG, Siegel G. Decreased prevalence of Alzheimer disease associated with 3-hydroxy-3-methyglutaryl coenzyme A reductase inhibitors. Arch Neurol 2000; 57:1439–1443.

199. Simons M, Keller P, Dichgans J, Schulz JB. Cholesterol and Alzheimer's disease. Neurology 2001; 57:1089–1093.

200. Hardy J, Selkoe DJ. Medicine – The amyloid hypothesis of Alzheimer's disease: Progress and problems on the road to therapeutics. Science 2002; 297:353–356.

201. Ritchie CW, Bush AI, Mackinnon A et al. Metal–protein attenuation with iodochlorhydroxyquin (clioquinol) targeting Abeta amyloid deposition and toxicity in Alzheimer disease: A pilot phase 2 clinical trial. Arch Neurol 2003; 60:1685–1691.

202. Selkoe D. The origins of Alzheimer disease: A is for amyloid. JAMA 2000; 283:1615–1617.

203. Esler WP, Wolfe MS. A portrait of Alzheimer secretases–New feature and familiar faces. Science 2001; 293:1449–1454.

204. Schenk D, Barbour R, Dunn K et al. Immunization with amyloid-ß attenuates Alzheimer-disease-like pathology in the PDAPP mouse. Nature 1999; 400:173–174.

205. Schenk DB, Seubert P, Liebergurg I, Wallace J. β-peptide immunization. A possible new treatment for Alzheimer disease. Arch Neurol 2000; 57:934–936.

206. Morgan D, Diamond DM, Gottschall PE et al. Aβ peptide vaccination prevents memory loss in an animal model of Alzheimer's disease. Nature 2000; 408:982–985.

207. Nicoll JAR, Wilkinson D, Holmes C et al. Neuropathology of human Alzheimer disease after immunization with amyloid-β-peptide: A case report. Nat Med 2003; 9:448–452.

208. Hock C, Konietzko U, Streffer JR et al. Antibodies against β-amyloid slow cognitive decline in Alzheimer's disease. Neuron 2003; 38:547–554.

209. DeMattos RB, Bales KR, Cummins DJ et al. Peripheral anti-Aβ antibody alters CNS and plasma Aβ clearance and decreases brain Aβ burden in a mouse model of Alzheimer's disease. Proc Natl Acad Sci U S A 2001; 98:8850–8855.

210. The Ronald and Nancy Reagan Research Institute of the Alzheimer's Association and the National Institute of Aging Work Group. Consensus report of the working group on molecular and biochemical markers of Alzheimer's disease. Neurobiol Aging 1998; 19:109–116.

211. Motter R, Vigo-Pelfrey C, Kholodenko D et al. Reduction of beta-amyloid peptide$_{42}$ in the cerebrospinal fluid of patients with Alzheimer's disease. Ann Neurol 1995; 38:643–648.

212. Galasko D, Chang L, Motter R et al. High cerebrospinal fluid tau and low amyloid-beta$_{42}$ levels in the clinical diagnosis of Alzheimer disease and relation to apolipoprotein e genotype. Arch Neurol 1998; 55:937–945.

213. Andreasen N, Vanmechelen E, Van de Voorde A et al. Cerebrospinal fluid tau protein as a biochemical marker for Alzheimer's disease: A community based follow up study. J Neurol Neurosurg Psychiatry 1998; 64:298–305.

214. Andreasen N, Minthon L, Davidsson P et al. Evaluation of CSF-tau and CSF-Aß$_{42}$ as diagnostic markers for Alzheimer disease in clinical practice. Arch Neurol 2001; 58:373–379.

215. American Psychiatric Association. Diagnostic and Statistical Manual of Mental Disorders. 4 edn. Washington, D.C.: American Psychiatric Association, 1994.

216. Hulstaert F, Blennow K, Ivanoiu A et al. Improved discrimination of AD patients using β-amyloid$_{(1–42)}$ and tau levels in CSF. Neurology 1999; 52:1555–1562.

217. Galasko D, Clark C, Chang L et al. Assessment of CSF levels of tau protein in mildly demented patients with Alzheimer's disease. Neurology 1997; 48:632–635.

218. Han X, Holtzman DM, McKeel DW, Jr., Kelley J, Morris JC. Substantial sulfatide deficiency and ceramide elevation in very early Alzheimer's disease: Potential role in disease pathogenesis. J Neurochem 2002; 82:809–818.

219. Han X, Holtzman DM, McKeel DW, Jr. Plasmalogen deficiency in early Alzheimer's disease subjects and in animal models: Molecular

characterization using electrospray ionization mass spectrometry. J Neurochem 2001; 77:1168–1180.

220. Han X, Fagan AM, Cheng H et al. Cerebrospinal fluid sulfatide is decreased in subjects with incipient dementia. Ann Neurol 2003; 54:115–119.

221. Han X, Cheng H, Fryer JD, Fagan AM, Holtzman DM. Novel role for apolipoprotein E in the central nervous system. Modulation of sulfatide content. J Biol Chem 2003; 278:8043.

222. World Health Organization. The ICD-10 classification of mental and behavioral disorders. Diagnostic criteria for research. Geneva: World Health Organization, 1993.

223. Teunissen CE, de Vente J, Steinbusch HW, De Bruijn C. Biochemical markers related to Alzheimer's dementia in serum and cerebrospinal fluid. Neurobiol Aging 2002; 23:485–508.

224. Lovell MA, Markesbery WR. Ratio of 8-hydroxyguanine in intact DNA to free 8-hydroxyguanine is increased in Alzheimer disease ventricular cerebrospinal fluid. Arch Neurol 2001; 58:392–396.

225. Fukumoto H, Tennis M, Locascio JJ et al. Age but not diagnosis is the main predictor of plasma amyloid β-protein levels. Arch Neurol 2003; 60:958–964.

226. DeMattos RB, Bales KR, Cummins DJ, Paul SM, Holtzman DM. Brain to plasma amyloid-β efflux: A measure of brain amyloid burden in a mouse model of Alzheimer's disease. Science 2002; 295:2264–2267.

227. Sperling RA, Sandson TA, Johnson KA. Functional imaging in Alzheimer's disease. In: Scinto LFM, Daffner KR, editors. Early Diagnosis of Alzheimer's Disease. Totowa, NJ: Humana Press, Inc., 2000: 149–168.

228. Vogt BA, Finch DM, Olson CR. Functional heterogeneity in cingulate cortex: The anterior executive and posterior evaluative regions. Cereb Cortex 1992; 2:435–443.

229. Braak H, Braak E. Neuropathological stageing of Alzheimer-related changes. Acta Neuropathol (Berl) 1991; 82:239–259.

230. Perani D, Bressi S, Cappa SF et al. Evidence of multiple memory systems in the human brain. A [18F]FDG PET metabolic study. Brain 1993; 116 (Pt 4):903–919.

231. Reed LJ, Marsden P, Lasserson D et al. FDG-PET analysis and findings in amnesia resulting from hypoxia. Memory 1999; 7:599–612.

232. Aupee AM, Desgranges B, Eustache F et al. Voxel-based mapping of brain hypometabolism in permanent amnesia with PET. Neuroimage 2001; 13:1164–1173.

233. Meguro K, Blaizot X, Kondoh Y et al. Neocortical and hippocampal glucose hypometabolism following neurotoxic lesions of the entorhinal and perirhinal cortices in the non-human primate as shown by PET: Implications for Alzheimer's disease. Brain 1999; 122:1519–1531.

234. Millien I, Blaizot X, Giffard C et al. Brain glucose hypometabolism after perirhinal lesions in baboons: Implications for Alzheimer disease and aging. J Cereb Blood Flow Metab 2002; 22:1248–1261.

235. Andreasen NC, O'Leary DS, Cizadlo T et al. II. PET studies of memory: Novel versus practiced free recall of word lists. Neuroimage 1995; 2:296–305.

236. Cabeza R, Nyberg L. Imaging Cognition II: An empirical review of 275 PET and fMRI studies. J Cogn Neurosci 2000; 12:1–47.

237. Maddock RJ. The retrosplenial cortex and emotion: New insights from functional neuroimaging of the human brain. Trends Neurosci 1999; 22:310–316.

238. Valenstein E, Bowers D, Verfaellie M et al. Retrosplenial amnesia. Brain 1987; 110:1631–1646.

239. Kennedy AM, Frackowiak RSJ, Newman SK et al. Deficits in cerebral glucose metabolism demonstrated by positron emission tomography in individuals at risk of familial Alzheimer's disease. Neurosci Lett 1995; 186:17–20.

240. Reiman EM, Caselli RJ, Yun LS et al. Preclinical evidence of Alzheimer's disease in persons homozygous for the epsilon 4 allele for apolipoprotein E. N Engl J Med 1996; 334:752–758.

241. Bookheimer SY, Strojwas MH, Cohen MS et al. Patterns of brain activation in people at risk for Alzheimer's disease. N Engl J Med 2000; 343:450–456.

242. Smith CD, Andersen AH, Kryscio RJ et al. Altered brain activation in cognitively intact individuals at high risk for Alzheimer's disease. Neurology 1999; 53:1391–1396.

243. Lustig C, Snyder AZ, Bhakta M et al. Functional deactivations: Change with age and dementia of the Alzheimer type. Proc Natl Acad Sci USA 2003; 100:14504–14509.

244. Zhuang ZP, Kung M-P, Hou C et al. Radioiodinated styrylbenzenes and thioflavins as probes for amyloid aggregates. J Med Chem 2001; 44:1905–1914.

245. Skovronsky DM, Zhang B, Kung MP et al. In vivo detection of amyloid plaques in a mouse model of Alzheimer's disease. Proc Natl Acad Sci U S A 2000; 97:7609–7614.

246. Klunk WE, Engler H, Nordberg A, et al. Imaging brain amyloid in Alzheimer's disease with Pittsburgh Compound-B. Ann Neurol. 2004; 55:306–319

247. Corder E, Saunders A, Strittmatter W et al. Gene dose of apolipoprotein E type 4 allele and the risk of Alzheimer's disease in late onset families. Science 1993; 261:921–923.

248. Mayeux RH, Saunders AM, Shea S et al. Utility of the apolipoprotein E genotype in the diagnosis of Alzheimer's disease. N Engl J Med 1998; 338:506–511.

249. Price JL, Ko AI, Wade MJ et al. Neuron number in the entorhinal cortex and CA1 in preclinical Alzheimer disease. Arch Neurol 2001; 58:1395–1402.

250. Tangalos EG, Smith GE, Ivnik RJ et al. The Mini-Mental State Examination in general medical practice: clinical utility and acceptance. Mayo Clin Proc 1996; 71:829–837.

251. Juva K, Sulkava R, Erkinjuntti T et al. Usefulness of the Clinical Dementia Rating scale in screening for dementia. Int Psychogeriatr 1995; 7:17–24.

252. Fuh JL, Teng EL, Lin KN et al. The Informant Questionnaire on Cognitive Decline in the Elderly (IQCODE) as a screening tool for dementia for a predominantly illiterate Chinese population. Neurology 1995; 45:92–96.

253. Rogers SL, Farlow MR, Doody RS et al. A 24-week, double-blind, placebo-controlled trial of donepezil in patients with Alzheimer's disease. Neurology 1998; 50:136–145.

254. Burns A, Rossor M, Hecker J et al. The effects of donepezil in Alzheimer's disease - results from a multinational trial. Dement Geriatr Cogn Disord 1999; 10:237–244.

255. Tariot PN, Solomon PR, Morris JC et al. A 5-month, randomized, placebo-controlled trial of galantamine in AD. Neurology 2000; 54:2269-2276.

256. Ellison L, Love S (eds) Neuropathology. London: Mosby, 1998

257. Danysz et al. Neuroprotective and symptomatological action of memantine relevant for Alzheimer's disease – a unified glutamatergic hypothesis on the mechanism of action. Neurotox Res 2000; 2:85–97.

258. Shumaker SA, Legault C, Kuller L et al. Conjugated equine estrogens and incidence of dementia and mild cognitive impairment in post-menopausal women: Women's Health Initiative Memory Study. JAMA 2004; 291:2947–2958.

Index

Please note: page numbers in *italics* refer to material in tables or boxes; those in **bold** type refer to figures.

acetylcholine, brain deficit 73-4, **75**
acetylcholinesterase inhibitors *see* cholinesterase inhibitors
activities of daily living (ADL)
    AD 36-7, 39–41
        case studies 105, 107, 110, 115
        dementia staging 49, *50, 52,* 67
        MCI 5–15
            AD subset 65–8, 105–8
            case studies 111, 112–14, 115, 117
AD *see* Alzheimer's disease
aging
    AD incidence 1–3
    brain atrophy 95–6
    cognitive changes, concepts 7, *10*
    cognitive performance 11–15
    comorbidity with AD 58
    memory impairment 3, *10*
        early treatment 69–71
    neuropathology 17–34
    non-demented
        case study 118–22
        dementia screening tests 44–9
        neuropathology 27–31
    normal cognitive decline 1–15
    plaques 25–31
    plasma Aβ levels 94
alpha-tocopherol *see* vitamin E
Alzheimer's disease (AD)
    brain hypometabolism 97
    comorbidity 58
    diagnostic criteria 37–8
        post-mortem 24–31
    early
        brain activity patterns 98–100
        case study 105–10
        cognitive tests 44–5
        detection 34, 35–52, 65–8
        staging 49, *50*
        symptoms 39–41

    early-onset 90, 101–3
    familial 90, 101–4
    genetic testing 90, 101–4
    inflammation in 93
    late-onset 90, 103–4
    MRI volumetrics 95
    neuropathology 17–34
    oxidative stress and 93
    prevalence 1–3
    progression to 6–10, 32, 65–8
        case study 110–17
        prevention 69–71
    rate of decline 13, 14–15
    risk factors 10, 54
    treatments
        cholinesterase inhibitors 75–80
        early stages 69–75
        under investigation 81–4
    vascular dementia and 59–60
Alzheimer's disease (AD) prodrome 57
amnestic MCI
    criteria 5, 6
    development of AD 55, *57*
    see also memory complaints
amyloid accumulation, control of 81–4
amyloid hypothesis 85–7
amyloid plaques 17–18, **19, 21**
    aging and NFT development 27
    imaging 90, 100–1
    inflammation in 93
    non-demented aging 27–31
    post-mortem 24–31
    progression of **22, 23,** 24, **25**
amyloid precursor protein (APP) 86–7, 91
amyloid precursor protein (*APP*) gene 90, 102, *103*
    mutations **85,** 87
amyloid vaccine 88–9

amyloid-beta peptide (Aβ) 85–7
    AD genes and 102, *103*, 104
    amyloid hypothesis 85–9
    biomarker *90, 91*
    CSF levels *90*, 91–2
    deposition 18–21, 24
    plasma levels 94
    protection against 81–4
anti-inflammatory agents *70*, 83, 93
anticholinergics 55
antioxidants *70*, 81
anxiety, cognitive complaints *4*
aphasia 41–2
    non-fluent 61, *64*
    semantic *41, 42*, 61, *64*
apolipoprotein E (*ApoE*) gene *90*, 103–4
apraxia *41*, 42
Aricept (donepezil) 77–8

basal forebrain, cholinergic cell loss 73,
    74
behavioural dysfunction 60–1
benign senescent forgetfulness 3, *10*
benzothiole amyloid agent 100–1
beta-amyloid protein (Aβ) *see* amyloid-
    beta peptide (Aβ)
biomarkers
    ideals for 89
    potential 89–94
brain
    hypometabolism 34, 97
    lesions *4*, 55
    structural imaging *90*, 95–6
butyrylcholinesterase 78

care, planning for 3
CDR (clinical dementia rating) 49, *50*
celebrex *70*
cerebrospinal fluid (CSF), biomarkers
    89–94
cerebrovascular disease *4*
chelation therapy 84
cholesterol-reducing agents 83
    trials *70*

cholinergic drugs, trials *70*
cholinergic hypothesis 73–5
cholinesterase inhibitors 75–80
    cost-effectiveness 76–7
    early use 69, 70–1
clinical dementia rating (CDR) 49, *50*
clioquinol 84
clock-drawing test 46–8
cognitive decline
    differential diagnosis 55, *56*
    early treatment 69–71
    informant-based history 39–41
    progressive 64–7
cognitive impairment
    fluctuations in 58, *59*
    mild *see* mild cognitive impairment
        (MCI)
    no dementia *10*
    rating 49, *50*
    reversible *4*
    screening 44–5
cognitive performance, aging and
    1–15
collateral information 37, 39–41
    AD early stages 105–9
    AD progression 110–17
    bias 118–22
    MCI progression 65–7
    value of 7
comorbidity 41, 43
    age-related disorders 58
    brain lesions 43, 55
computed tomography (CT)
    lesions in dementia 42–3
    structural imaging 33, 95
confrontation naming 11
cortical hypoperfusion 34
corticobasal degeneration *41, 42*, 55, *57*
Creutzfeldt-Jakob disease *41, 42, 57*

daily living activities *see* activities of
    daily living (ADL)
dementia
    cholinesterase inhibitors 77
    definition *36*

early 35–6
    case study 110–17
early-onset 61
features 41–2
frontotemporal lobar 60–5, **66–7**
hallmarks *37*
long-term assessment 46–9
MRI imaging 42–3
neuropsychiatric symptoms 32
normal aging and 1–3
Parkinson's 42
progressive, case study 105–9
risk, brain metabolic deficits 98
risk reduction 71–3
screening instruments 45–9
semantic 60
staging 49–51
treatment 73–84
vascular 4, *57*, 59–60, *61*
dementia with Lewy bodies (DLB)
58, *59*
    differential diagnosis *41, 42,*
        55, 57
    MCI in 4
dementia prodrome 2–3, *4*
    aging 11, 15–16
    depression 54
depression
    cognitive complaints 4
    cognitive defects and 43
    memory complaints 54
diagnosis
    dementia 36–45
    early AD 35–45
    future strategies 85–104
    MCI 36–45
        differential diagnosis 53–67
    neuroimaging *90*, 95–101
DLB *see* dementia with Lewy bodies
    (DLB)
donepezil *70*, 75–8
    combination therapy 80
    early AD 106
driving difficulty
    case study 106, 107, 108, 112, 117
    diagnosis *39, 40, 49, 65*

entorhinal cortex
    AD defects **22, 23**
    atrophy 96
    MCI changes 31
    plaques 18, **19**
episodic memory 11
estrogen 81–2
    trials *70*
Exelon (rivastigmine) 78
extrapyramidal signs *41, 42*

familial disorders
    AD *38*
        brain activity changes 98–100
        genetic testing 101–4
        or normal aging, case study
          118–22
    FTDs 61
families
    care planning 3
    see also collateral information
focal neurological deficits 42
forgetfulness
    aging 1–15
    worried well 53
frontotemporal dementia 4
frontotemporal lobar degeneration 42,
    55, 57
frontotemporal lobar dementias
    (FTDs) 60–5, **66–7**
functional neuroimaging *90*, 96–101

gait, abnormal *41*, 42
galactocerebrosides (sulfatides) *90*, 92–3
galantamine 78–9
    early AD case history 107
    hypothetical response to **72**
    trial **72**
GDS (global deterioration scale) 50–1
genetic risk factors 32
genetic testing *90*, 101–4
ginko biloba *70*, 107
global deterioration scale (GDS) 50–1
glutamate receptor blocker 79–80

glutamatergic drugs, trials 70
Hachinski Ischemic Score (modified) 60, 61
hallucinations 32, 58, 59
hippocampus
   atrophy 96
   defects in AD **22**, **23**, *31*
   imaging 33–4
   neuron loss 19–21, **22**
   structural imaging 90
history
   cognitive decline 65–8
   see also collateral information
hormone replacement therapy 81–2

ibuprofen *70*, 83
imaging
   amyloid plaques *90*, 100–1
   diagnostic *90*, 95–101
   functional *90*, 96–101
   radiological evaluation in AD 42–3
   structural *90*, 95–6
   techniques 32–4
immunization strategies 88–9
infectious diseases 55, *56*
inflammation markers *90*, 93
informant *see* collateral information; self-reported memory loss
insight, MCI and 111, 114, 117
items mislaid *see* misplacement of items

language difficulty 41–2
   worried well 53
leisure activities
   decline in performance 40, 106, 111
   mental stimulation 71–3
Lewy bodies, with dementia *see* dementia with Lewy bodies (DLB)
lipid peroxidation 93–4

magnetic resonance imaging (MRI)
   functional (fMRI) *90*, 98–100
   hippocampus morphology 33

lesions in dementia 42–3
   structural imaging *90*, 95–6
magnetic resonance spectroscopy (MRS) 33
MCI *see* mild cognitive impairment
medial temporal lobe
   functional imaging 97, 100
   loss 33
   structural imaging 96
medication
   for AD / MCI *see* treatment
   cognitive effects 4, 55, *56*, 72
memantine 79–80
memory complaints
   non-demented aging 118–22
   self-reported 39
   see also amnestic MCI
memory loss
   AD-associated 41, 42, 44
   age-associated 3–5, *10*, 11
   brain functional imaging 97
   dementia-associated *36*, 37
   MCI-associated 5–7, 8–9, 39, *41*
   screening for 45, 46–9, *50–2*
   self-reported 53–4
      progression to AD 110–17
   short term, case study 105–6, 108
memory tasks, fMRI 98–9
mental status testing 44–5
mental stimulation 71–3
mild cognitive impairment (MCI)
   AD subset 65–8
   brain hypometabolism 98
   conversion to AD 6–10, 32
      prevention 69–71
   definitions 3–5
   detection 35–52
   differential diagnosis 53–67
   early AD, case study 105–10
   early symptoms 39–41
   forms of *57*
   medial temoporal lobe atrophy 96
   neuropathology 31–4
   progression of, case study 110–17
   treatment 69–80
mild neurocognitive decline *10*

mini-mental state examination (MMSE)
44, 45–6, 47
cognitive performance, case study
104
MCI criteria 5, 6
misplacement of items
AD case study 108, 109, 114, 115,
121
AD diagnosis 40
MMSE see mini-mental state
examination (MMSE)
molecular imaging, amyloid plaques
100–1
monoamine oxidase inhibitor 81
monoclonal Aβ antibodies 94
movement disorder 42
MRI see magnetic resonance imaging
(MRI)
MRS (magnetic resonance spectroscopy) 33
myoclonus 41

N-methyl-D-aspartate (NMDA)
glutamte receptor blocker 79–80
neural activity, fMRI 98–9
neurodegenerative dementias 55,
56, 57
neurofibrillary tangles (NFTs) 17,
18–19, 20, 21
aging and 27
oxidative stress 93
progression 22–4, 25
tau in 91
neurogenetic disorders 56
neuroimaging 42–3
see also imaging
neurological examination 37, 41–2
neurons
loss
AD 19–21, 30
MCI 31–2
Pick's disease 64
in non-demented aging 29
neuropsychiatric symptoms 32,
58, 59
nicotinic receptor agonist 78–9

NMDA (N-methyl-D-aspartate)
glutamte receptor blocker 79–80
non-pharmacological treatment
71–3

operationalized amnestic MCI 6
oxidative stress markers 90, 93–4

Parkinsonism 41, 42
Parkinson's disease
biomarkers 94
comorbidity 58
personal care, early AD 106, 107
physical activity, benefits 71–3
Pick's disease 57, 64
Pittsburgh compound-B (PIB) 100–1
plaques see amyloid plaques; senile
plaques
positron emission tomography (PET)
33, 34, 43
amyloid tracer 100–1
functional imaging 90, 96–8
presenilin genes (Ps-1/Ps-2) 90,
102–3
prion disorders 41, 42, 57
prodromal AD 57
prodromal dementia see dementia
prodrome
progressive non-fluent aphasia 61, 64
pseudo-dementia 54
psychiatric symptoms 32, 58, 59
psychometric testing 44–5
psychomotor speed 11

Razadyne 70, 75–7, 78–9
repetition
AD
case study 108, 109, 114,
115, 121
diagnosis 40, 41
frontotemporal lobar degeneration
64
reversible cognitive dysfunction 4
rivastigmine 70, 75–7, 78

screening tests 45–9
secretase inhibitors 87–8
selegiline 81
selenium *70*
self-reported memory loss 7, 53–4
semantic aphasia *41*, 42, 61, *64*
semantic dementia 60
senile plaques 17, 18, 24–5, **26**
  oxidative stress 93
serum biomarkers *90*, 94
seven-minute screen 48–9
sexually transmitted diseases 43, 55, *56*
single-photon emission computed
  tomography (SPECT) 33, 34, 43
  functional imaging *90*, 96–8
speech disorder
  FTDs 60–1
  see also aphasia
staging tests 49–50, *51–2*
statins 83
structural neuroimaging *90*, 95–6
suicide 112, 117
sulfatide *90*, 92–3
syphilis 43

tacrine 75
tau gene abnormalities 64

tau protein **17**, 18–19, **20**, **21**, **25**
  biomarker *90*, 91–2
thyroid disorders 43, *56*
treatment
  AD 80–4
  dementia 73–80
  future strategies 85–104
  MCI 69–73
  non-pharmacological 71–3

vascular dementia 4, *57*, 59–60, *61*
vascular disease
  comorbidity 58
  focal neurological deficits 42
visual field deficit 42
visual memory 5
visuospatial ability 11
vitamin B12, deficiency 43, *56*
vitamin C 81
vitamin E *70*, 81
  in early AD case history 105, 107

worried well 4, 53–4
  memory complaints 39